Aging in Place: Designing, Adapting, and Enhancing the Home Environment

Aging in Place: Designing, Adapting, and Enhancing the Home Environment has been co-published simultaneously as *Physical & Occupational Therapy in Geriatrics,* Volume 16, Numbers 3/4 1999.

The *Physical & Occupational Therapy in Geriatrics* Monographic "Separates"

Below is a list of "separates," which in serials librarianship means a special issue simultaneously published as a special journal issue or double-issue *and* as a "separate" hardbound monograph. (This is a format which we also call a "DocuSerial.")

"Separates" are published because specialized libraries or professionals may wish to purchase a specific thematic issue by itself in a format which can be separately cataloged and shelved, as opposed to purchasing the journal on an on-going basis. Faculty members may also more easily consider a "separate" for classroom adoption.

"Separates" are carefully classified separately with the major book jobbers so that the journal tie-in can be noted on new book order slips to avoid duplicate purchasing.

You may wish to visit Haworth's website at . . .

http://www.haworthpressinc.com

. . . to search our online catalog for complete tables of contents of these separates and related publications.

You may also call 1-800-HAWORTH (outside US/Canada: 607-722-5857), or Fax 1-800-895-0582 (outside US/Canada: 607-771-0012), or e-mail at:

getinfo@haworthpressinc.com

Aging in Place: Designing, Adapting, and Enhancing the Home Environment, edited by Ellen D. Taira, OTR/L, MPH, and Jodi L. Carlson, MS, OTR/L (Vol. 16, No. 3/4, 1999). *This important book examines the current trends in adaptive home designs for older adults and explores innovative home designs and studies for creating environments that offer optimal living for aging adults.*

The Mentally Impaired Elderly: Strategies and Interventions to Maintain Function, edited by Ellen D. Taira, OTR/L, MPH (Vol. 9, No. 3/4, 1991). *"Caregivers will benefit from this book as it provides information on methods and strategies to deal with mentally impaired elderly patients."* (Senior News)

Aging in the Designed Environment, edited by Margaret A. Christenson, MPH, OTR (Vol. 8, No. 3/4, 1990). *"Presents the environment as the untapped treatment modality that can maximize a person's functional abilities when designed effectively. . . . integrates theory with practice to provide a very coherent and stimulating book."* (Canadian Journal of Occupational Therapy)

Successful Models of Community Long Term Care Services for the Elderly, edited by Eloise H. P. Killeffer, EdM, and Ruth Bennett, PhD (Vol. 8, No. 1/2, 1990). *"Provides invaluable information to practitioners, educators, policymakers, and researchers concerned with meeting the myriad needs of the elderly."* (Patricia A. Miller, MEd, OTR, FAOTA, Assistant Professor of Clinical Occupational Therapy and Public Health, Columbia University)

Assessing the Driving Ability of the Elderly: A Preliminary Investigation, edited by Ellen D. Taira, OTR/L, MPH (Vol. 7, No. 1/2, 1989). *" 'The' resource for older driver assessment. This new book provides a review of older driver literature, guidelines for practitioners who must assess older driver skills, and offers twenty-one screening instruments that test the visual, motor, and cognitive abilities of mature drivers."* (Resources in Aging)

Promoting Quality Long Term Care for Older Persons, edited by Ellen D. Taira, OTR/L, MPH (Vol. 6, No. 3/4, 1989). *Exciting programs in long term care–designed to better serve elderly persons with chronic diseases–are highlighted in this rich volume.*

Rehabilitation Interventions for the Institutionalized Elderly, edited by Ellen D. Taira, OTR/L, MPH (Vol. 6, No. 2, 1989). *"A sample of rehabilitation interventions which, combined in this volume, provide a holistic approach to gerontic services for those who are institutionalized."* (Advances for Occupational Therapists)

Community Programs for the Health Impaired Elderly, edited by Ellen D. Taira, OTR/L, MPH (Vol. 6, No. 1, 1989). *"This is an easy-to-read reference book occupational therapists can use to explore and develop techniques and programs to meet individual and community needs."* (American Journal of Occupational Therapists)

Community Programs for the Depressed Elderly: A Rehabilitation Approach, edited by Ellen D. Taira, OTR/L, MPH (Vol. 5, No. 1, 1987). *"A timely publication as recognition of the serious magnitude of depression amongst the elderly continues to grow." (Canadian Journal of Occupational Therapy)*

Therapeutic Interventions for the Person with Dementia, edited by Ellen D. Taira, OTR/L, MPH (Vol. 4, No. 3, 1986). *"Packed with useful information. The reader gains a better grasp of the patience, understanding, and flexibility needed to help these people. This is excellent reading for therapists and students and a valuable addition to the library of anyone working with the elderly." (American Journal of Occupational Therapy)*

Handbook of Innovative Programs for the Impaired Elderly, edited by Eloise H. P. Killeffer, EdM, Ruth Bennett, PhD, and Gerta Gruen, MPH (Vol. 3, No. 3, 1985). *"A handy source of ideas for promoting maintenance of physical abilities, restoring physical and mental abilities, and linking residents with organizations and services in the surrounding community and opening the long-term care facility to the community." (Canadian Journal of Occupational Therapy)*

A Handbook of Assistive Devices for the Handicapped Elderly: New Help for Independent Living, by Joseph M. Breuer, MA, RPT (Vol. 1, No. 2, 1982). *"Practical advice is coupled with a significant theoretical background and valuable experience." (Journal of the American Geriatrics Society)*

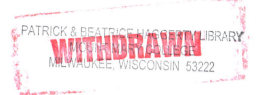
Aging in Place:
Designing, Adapting,
and Enhancing
the Home Environment

Ellen D. Taira, OTR/L, MPH
Jodi L. Carlson, MS, OTR/L
Editors

Aging in Place: Designing, Adapting, and Enhancing the Home Environment has been co-published simultaneously as *Physical & Occupational Therapy in Geriatrics,* Volume 16, Numbers 3/4 1999.

The Haworth Press, Inc.
New York • London • Oxford

Aging in Place: Designing, Adapting, and Enhancing the Home Environment has been co-published simultaneously as *Physical & Occupational Therapy in Geriatrics,* Volume 16, Numbers 3/4 1999.

The development, preparation, and publication of this work has been undertaken with great care. However, the publisher, employees, editors, and agents of The Haworth Press and all imprints of The Haworth Press, Inc., including The Haworth Medical Press® and Pharmaceutical Products Press®, are not responsible for any errors contained herein or for consequences that may ensue from use of materials or information contained in this work. Opinions expressed by the author(s) are not necessarily those of The Haworth Press, Inc.

The Haworth Press, Inc., 10 Alice Street, Binghamton, NY 13904-1580 USA

Cover design by Thomas J. Mayshock Jr.

Library of Congress Cataloging-in-Publication Data

Aging in place: designing, adapting, and enhancing the home environment / Ellen D. Taira, Jodi L. Carlson. editors.
      p. cm.
      "Aging in place: designing, adapting, and enhancing the home environment has been co-published simultaneously as Physical & occupational therapy in geriatrics, volume 16, numbers 3/4 1999."
      Includes bibliographical references and index.
      ISBN 0-7890-0971-4 (alk. paper) – ISBN 0-7890-0989-7 (alk. paper)
      1. Architecture and the aged. I. Taira, Ellen D. II. Carlson, Jodi L.

NA2545.A3 A35 2000
720'.84'6–dc21

                                     00-021099

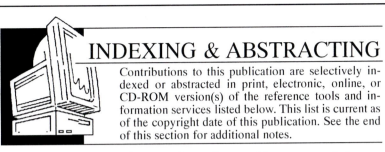

INDEXING & ABSTRACTING

Contributions to this publication are selectively indexed or abstracted in print, electronic, online, or CD-ROM version(s) of the reference tools and information services listed below. This list is current as of the copyright date of this publication. See the end of this section for additional notes.

- *Abstracts in Social Gerontology: Current Literature on Aging*
- *Academic Abstracts/CD-ROM*
- *AgeInfo CD-Rom*
- *Alzheimer's Disease Education & Referral Center (ADEAR)*
- *Brown University Geriatric Research Application Digest "Abstracts Section"*
- *BUBL Information Service: An Internet-based Information Service for the UK higher education community <URL: http://bubl.ac.uk/>*
- *CINAHL (Cumulative Index to Nursing & Allied Health Literature)*
- *CNPIEC Reference Guide: Chinese National Directory of Foreign Periodicals*
- *EMBASE/Excerpta Medica Secondary Publishing Division*
- *Family Studies Database (online and CD/ROM)*
- *Health Source: Indexing & Abstracting of 160 selected health related journals, updated monthly: EBSCO Publishing*
- *Health Source Plus: expanded version of "Health Source:" EBSCO Publishing*
- *Human Resources Abstracts (HRA)*
- *MANTIS (Manual, Alternative & Natural Therapy)*
- *New Literature on Old Age*
- *Occupational Therapy Database (OTDBASE)*
- *Occupational Therapy Index*
- *OT BibSys*

(continued)

- *PAIS (Public Affairs Information Service) NYC www.pais.org*
- *Psychological Abstracts (PsycINFO)*
- *REHABDATA, National Rehabilitation Information Center*
- *Social Work Abstracts*
- *SPORTDiscus*

*Special Bibliographic Notes related to special journal issues
(separates) and indexing/abstracting:*

- indexing/abstracting services in this list will also cover material in any "separate" that is co-published simultaneously with Haworth's special thematic journal issue or DocuSerial. Indexing/abstracting usually covers material at the article/chapter level.

- monographic co-editions are intended for either non-subscribers or libraries which intend to purchase a second copy for their circulating collections.

- monographic co-editions are reported to all jobbers/wholesalers/approval plans. The source journal is listed as the "series" to assist the prevention of duplicate purchasing in the same manner utilized for books-in-series.

- to facilitate user/access services all indexing/abstracting services are encouraged to utilize the co-indexing entry note indicated at the bottom of the first page of each article/chapter/contribution.

- this is intended to assist a library user of any reference tool (whether print, electronic, online, or CD-ROM) to locate the monographic version if the library has purchased this version but not a subscription to the source journal.

- individual articles/chapters in any Haworth publication are also available through the Haworth Document Delivery Service (HDDS).

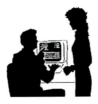

Aging in Place:
Designing, Adapting, and Enhancing the Home Environment

CONTENTS

ABOUT THE EDITORS

Ellen Dunleavey Taira, OTR/L, MPH, is Manager of the Rehabilitation Department in the Home Health Agency of Montefiore Medical Center, The University Hospital for the Albert Einstein College of Medicine, Bronx, New York. She is a doctoral student in social gerontology at Fordham University. She has taught gerontology to Master's students in occupational therapy in several programs in New York City. Throughout her career, Ms. Taira has provided her expertise, as an occupational therapist and a gerontologist, in a variety of community and institutional settings. She has worked as a case manager and researcher in a home health and day health program in San Francisco. In her work as a program specialist in long-term care for the state of Hawaii, she assisted in the development of programs to serve the socially and economically needy elderly, compiled the first directory of long-term care services in Hawaii, and promoted the integration of services for the disabled and elderly.

Ms. Taira has served on numerous boards and committees to expand community-based services. She has written extensively on the subject of long-term care, presented papers at national conferences, and acted as spokesperson for the needs of the elderly disabled in many settings.

Jodi L. Carlson, MS, OTR/L, is a private practitioner in Westchester and Putnam counties in the state of New York. She works in adult homes for the developmentally disabled, works for Westchester and Putnam Hospice, and participates in research on developing occupational therapy programs for community settings. Ms. Carlson has practiced as an occupational therapist for six years.

Foreword

A year ago I took my 84 year old mother to a marvelous Broadway play, *The Beauty Queen of Lenane*, about an extremely troublesome example of aging in place in Ireland. In an effort to accommodate her failing hearing (she refuses an aide), I selected expensive mezzanine seats where you could see and hear perfectly. Alas, it involved a long torturous trek down steps without a railing. Mother refused to try the steps even with the help of several people and was placed in a chair at the top of the stairs. I noted with chagrin that the beautiful turn of the century theater had recently been renovated. But of course, there was no need for a railing, because where would you put it? Its intrusive, not to mention unsightly appearance, would block the entrance to the seats of others.

The story has a happy ending because the compassionate manager of the theater was informed of the situation and we were led to some empty seats near the very front of the orchestra by a helpful usher. Accommodation certainly, but not the kind discussed in this volume.

For the past year the idea of a special volume on *Aging in Place* has enticed me. First, the Smithsonian's design museum in New York, the Cooper-Hewitt, organized an exhibit on universal design, bringing the subject into the mainstream. Around the same time, a one day conference in New York, sponsored by the Pride Institute, called Aging and the Home Environment: Enhancing the Care through Design, piqued my interest. The enormously responsive multidisciplinary audience was enthralled with the suggestions offered by the design experts. Clearly, this was a subject that crossed many discipline boundaries because everyone was committed to continued community living.

Universal design is about inclusion, perhaps a natural progression of the last 25 years of efforts to include the disabled in the mainstream of American life. First, there was section 504.c in 1974 which mandated accessible features like curb cuts and tactile numbers on eleva-

[Haworth indexing entry note]: "Foreword." Taira, Ellen D. Published in *Aging in Place: Designing, Adapting, and Enhancing the Home Environment* (ed: Ellen D. Taira, and Jodi L. Carlson) The Haworth Press, Inc. 1999, pp. xiii-xiv. Single or multiple copies of this article are available for a fee from The Haworth Document Delivery Service [1-800-342-9678, 9:00 a.m. - 5:00 p.m. (EST). E-mail address: getinfo@haworth pressinc.com].

xiii

tors in publicly funded buildings. Later, the Americans with Disabilities Act (ADA) addressed workplace issues which required employers to consider universal design when determining the height of file cabinets, for example, or allowing a wheelchair user access to files. ADA legislation continues to influence and support design for inclusion and accessibility, both in the workplace and at home. In addition to the timeliness and appeal of the aging in place theme, this volume is unusual because of the diversity of the contributors. No rehabilitation professional would doubt the important role in rehabilitation research for architects and universal design specialists but they have only lately found a place in the mainstream.

Contributors for this volume all speak to larger issues like placement of furniture and handrails as well as sophisticated design concepts such as Jon Sanford and colleagues' marvelous discussion of adaptations for toilets and how ADA guidelines do not meet the needs of older adults. Larry Trachtman and colleagues present original thinking for every room in the house, essential to allow us to think "out of the box." Susan Klein and colleagues in Philadelphia speak to the housing/rehab connection at an area agency on aging, sadly an uncommon occurrence, even as we approach the millennium.

On a more global level, Phoebe Liebig gives a fascinating account of care for the aged in India, which, although unlike anything we know, does indeed speak to adapting and making due with what is on hand in a way that should prompt us to think about aging in place from a traditional perspective. Cynthia Stuen and Roxane Offner's overview of vision loss is essential reading for anyone who comes in contact with elderly clients or consumers including aging theater goers as noted above. The list of vision rehab resources is especially helpful.

Cream and Teaford surveyed aged persons' use of telephone modifications, surely an excellent example of an industry that adopted universal design concepts like large button phones long before it was fashionable.

Auriemma and colleagues present an overview of current knowledge important to professionals involved in adaptive home design. Pat Crist did a qualitative study on the effect of housing type on whether housing type affected the quality of life of older persons. Not surprisingly, everyone prefers to age in place.

I hope you enjoy reading this volume as much as I have.

Ellen D. Taira
Editor

The Universal Design Home: Are We Ready for It?

Lawrence H. Trachtman, MS
Ronald L. Mace, BArch, FAIA
Leslie C. Young, MF
Rex J. Pace, DED

SUMMARY. Changes in who we are and what we can do require a world that is more accommodating to variances in mobility, vision, hearing, cognition, and manual dexterity. Universal design is an approach to creating everyday environments and products that are usable by all people to the greatest extent possible, regardless of age or ability. "The Next Generation Universal Home" is a concept design of ideal and desired universal design features in single-family housing. This paper illustrates ways to make our homes more universally usable, as well as providing rationale for a more universal approach to the design of our built environment. *[Article copies available for a fee from The Haworth Document Delivery Service: 1-800-342-9678. E-mail address: getinfo@haworth pressinc.com <Website: http://www.haworthpressinc.com>]*

Lawrence H. Trachtman, Leslie C. Young and Rex J. Pace are affiliated with The Center for Universal Design, School of Design, Box 8613, North Carolina State University, Raleigh, NC 27695-8613 (E-mail: trachtman@ncsu.edu). Ronald L. Mace (deceased, June 29, 1998) was also affiliated with The Center for Universal Design, School of Design, North Carolina University.

This work was supported in part under grant #H133E40003 from the National Institute on Disability and Rehabilitation Research of the U.S. Department of Education. The opinions expressed in this publication are those of the authors and do not necessarily reflect those of the U.S. Department of Education.

[Haworth co-indexing entry note]: "The Universal Design Home: Are We Ready for It?" Trachtman, Lawrence H. et al. Co-published simultaneously in *Physical & Occupational Therapy in Geriatrics* (The Haworth Press, Inc.) Vol. 16, No. 3/4, 1999, pp. 1-18; and: *Aging in Place: Designing, Adapting, and Enhancing the Home Environment* (ed: Ellen D. Taira, and Jodi L. Carlson) The Haworth Press, Inc., 1999, pp. 1-18. Single or multiple copies of this article are available for a fee from The Haworth Document Delivery Service [1-800-342-9678, 9:00 a.m. - 5:00 p.m. (EST). E-mail address: getinfo@haworthpressinc.com].

KEYWORDS. Universal design, accessible design, barrier-free design, life-span design, housing, disability, aging

INTRODUCTION

Universal design of environments and tools and objects of daily use is a concept or philosophy for design that recognizes, respects, values, and attempts to accommodate the broadest possible spectrum of human ability. It requires sensitivity to and knowledge about people of all ages and abilities. Sometimes referred to as lifespan design or transgenerational design, it encompasses and goes beyond the accessible, adaptable, and barrier free design concepts of the past. It helps eliminate the need for special features and spaces for people with disabilities which are often stigmatizing, embarrassing, different looking, and usually more expensive. Universal design is a marketing issue as well as a design concept since products and spaces that are more universally usable are marketable to nearly everyone. And, as more universally designed products become mass-produced, they become available at lower cost to all users, thus minimizing the need for special products or some assistive technology for persons with disabilities or older individuals.

Universal design is an approach to creating everyday environments and products (e.g., a level entrance, a lever door handle, rocker panel light switch) that are usable by all people to the greatest extent possible, regardless of age or ability (Mace, Hardie, & Place, 1991). As a result, universal design is neither an assistive technology (specialized device), nor is it a euphemism for accessible design (specialized product or environment). Rather, universal design involves a fundamental shift in thinking about accessibility away from the practice of removing or overcoming environmental barriers for an individual or particular group of people (i.e., those with disabilities) to a way of meeting the environmental needs of all users (Bednar, 1977).

Specialized design is predicated on the notion that people with functional limitations are different from people without such limitations and therefore require special products or technologies. Universal design, on the other hand, makes no such assumptions. On the contrary, universal design is *inclusive design*. It eliminates the distinction between people with disabilities and the rest of society. Universal design promotes design for children, older people, and people with disabilities without considering each as separate groups of users; it presumes that people comprise a continuum of needs and abilities. By increasing the number of people whose needs are being addressed, universal design presumes that one good solution that meets the needs of a broad range of users is more desirable, convenient, and economical as well as less stigmatizing than multiple solutions for a myriad of subpopulations (Sanford, Story & Ringholz, 1998). However, it is important to acknowledge that one good design solution for everyone is an ideal goal that may not always be achievable. As such, universal design is, in reality, an ongoing and iterative process through which the needs of ever increasing portions of the population can be met.

When well implemented, universal design can be invisible, marketable, profitable, safe, and both physically and emotionally accessible to most users. In simple terms, universal design is user-based "good design" carried somewhat beyond the narrowly focused but commonly accepted averages in human factors. It might be called "more inclusive user-based design" because it includes the abilities and needs of people who are beyond "average."

THE MOVEMENT TOWARD MORE UNIVERSAL DESIGN

Changes in who we are, what we can do, and where we live require a world that is more accommodating to variances in mobility, vision, hearing, cognition, and manual dexterity. People with disabilities are aging, and healthy people are also aging into disability. All aspects of the physical environment including building layout and elements, signage, signal and alarm systems, telecommunications, and other user interfaces will have to be redesigned to accommodate the needs of an increasing number of people with some type of limitation. In fact, the magnitude of the population shift suggests that it would make more sense to design products and environments for *everyone* rather than creating different designs specifically for individuals who have disabilities (Sanford, Story & Ringholz, 1998). This change in thinking underlies the movement toward universal design.

Universal design has its origins in both the disability and design communities. The disability community, frustrated by the lack of commercially available products, misconceptions of disability, and attitudinal barriers often fostered by specialized and stigmatizing design solutions, expects universal design to increase the prevalence of accessibility and usability in the built environment, as well as to enhance opportunities for participation and social integration of people with disabilities in everyday life (Mace, Hardie, & Place, 1991). Universal design has also found proponents among designers and social scientists who see it as a mechanism to achieve a more pluralistic definition of good design predicated on its responsiveness to the needs of users (Welch, 1995).

A Legislative Agenda

The disability rights movement that blossomed during the 1970s began a legislative agenda for accessibility that would later strengthen a movement for more universal design. Federal legislation such as the Rehabilitation Act of 1973 addressed issues that were important to the disability community. The power of the Rehabilitation Act is that its language, especially Section 504, echoes Title VII of the 1964 Civil Rights Act. Section 504 was the first statutory definition of discrimination towards people with disabilities. Although it did not have the scope of the Civil Rights Act of 1964, and only outlaws discrimination by those entities that receive federal funds, it was a crucial factor in shifting disability issues from the realm of social services and therapeutic practice to a political and civil rights context (Welch, 1995). Section 504 introduced the concept of program accessibility, which allowed programs to achieve accessibility by being "viewed in their entirety." This permitted some flexibility for compliance. For example, a community program could relocate activities to a physically accessible space in lieu of costly renovations to an existing location.

Today, accessibility has been given much impetus by the Fair Housing Act Amendments of 1988, the Americans with Disabilities Act of 1990, and now the Telecommunications Act of 1996. Universal design, however, goes far beyond minimum standards to include maximum or optimum features whenever possible. Thus, it eliminates labels that separate, stigmatize and cause general public or consumer market avoidance. Universal design is *not* a euphemism for accessibility. It is not a catchy phrase to make more palatable the requirements of the ADA Standards for Accessible Design. It is a term that re-establishes an important goal of good design–to meet the needs of as many users as possible. *Universal* indicates a unanimity of practice and applicability to all cases without significant exception (Welch, 1995). Universal design suggests solutions that are capable of being adjusted or modified to meet varied requirements. It is the inclusive nature of universal design that makes it cost effective. Universal design increases the number of people whose needs are being addressed and it encourages an integrative approach rather than multiple separate solutions (Welch, 1995).

Universal design is not an issue like "barrier free" or "adaptable" design which can be required by laws and for which prescriptive standards can be made enforceable. There are no standards or specifications that prescribe universal design. Since it is known that most of the features designed for people with disabilities are easier and safer for others to use, there is some guidance in the standards and specifications for accessible and adaptable design. There is similar limited guidance in the few specifications available on design for children and older people. Designers must abide by the mandated minimums of existing laws and standards, but also go beyond them to achieve universal design. Since the existing standards do not directly apply to all spaces and products, designers must also interpolate or interpret prescriptive requirements for application in other settings. More importantly, universal designers must compare the various sources of information with the experience and feedback of end users, study good examples, and be focused on the suitability of proposed design solutions, a demanding task for which many designers are not yet prepared and for whom much support and development is needed.

Benefits to People with Disabilities and Older Individuals

Although universal design is beneficial to all consumers, it is most needed by those who have a limitation. It may not be valued by those who do not have an immediate need even though later in life it may be perceived as beneficial and more valued. Promoting universal design for that future possibility may be perceived as negative, threatening, or stigmatizing and cause non-disabled consumers to shun it. Family members of aging parents also may not recognize the immediate benefits of universal design in housing or product choices.

Universal design is also lifespan design. All of us benefit from accessible places and products at many stages in the passage from childhood to old age. The case for universal design is frequently made by citing national census data and projections. In 1990, 48.9 million

Americans had some type of disability and 31 million, one in every eight Americans, were 65 or older; by 2030 it is predicted that one in five Americans will be over 65 (Welch, 1995). While statistics can be informative, designing for children, older people and people with disabilities is not thinking about separate groups of users but the spectrum of human-environment interaction.

People with disabilities and seniors benefit dramatically from the effective and early adoption of universal design by industry. Benefits include, but are not limited to the following:

- Availability of more usable consumer products at regular prices and from existing local commercial sources;
- Unprecedented accessibility to public and commercial facilities and services including recreation and communications;
- An improved image as customers and participants rather than patients, clients, or service recipients; and
- Greater choice in location, style, size, and cost of housing that may prevent relocation as abilities change over time.

Other consumers benefit from universal design through safer, more comfortable, and usable products and environments as well as the ability to confidently remain in place at times of temporary disability and as abilities diminish with age. Producers benefit from an expanded market for fewer products. Universal design improves independence, affordability, marketability, and user image and identity. It is a multidimensional and interdisciplinary issue that requires change in the knowledge, strategies, and procedures of designers, manufacturers, builders, and marketers in all industries.

UNIVERSAL DESIGN IN HOUSING

There are no requirements in the U.S. that single-family or other forms of private housing be accessible or barrier free, and there is little incentive for the housing industry to change. Most accessible housing is built by and for persons with disabilities on an individual basis. Very little accessible housing is available on the open market and housing opportunities for people with disabilities continue to be extremely limited. Realtors, citing stigma, largely discount accessible homes as not marketable to others and devalue them in the marketplace.

The idea for universal design in housing grew out of recognition that because most of the features needed by people with disabilities were useful to others, there was justification to make their inclusion common practice. For example, raising electrical receptacles to 15 inches or 18 inches above the floor eliminates the need to bend over as far and makes them easier for everyone, or more universal. Some universal features make common activities easier for all. For example, moving day is much easier in houses with stepless entrances and wider doors and hallways. Some universal design features create experiences many people have not had before. For example, when well designed, bathrooms with extra floor space to accommodate users of mobility aids are perceived as luxurious and people revel in their newfound ability to have furniture in the bathroom. A chair, bookcase, towel rack, or storage shelf can give bathrooms a marketable elegance. They can be removed if the space is ever needed to accommodate a family member or friend.

Universal design in housing far exceeds the minimum specifications of legislated barrier free and accessible mandates. Universal design in housing applies universal design principles to all spaces, features, and aspects of houses and creates homes that are usable by and marketable to people of all ages and abilities. Some features of universally designed homes are adjustable to meet particular needs or needs that change as family members age, yet allow the home to remain marketable. Universal design has the unique quality that when done well it is invisible.

The Next Generation Universal Home

"The Next Generation Universal Home" is one of the last projects that Ron Mace worked on before his passing in June 1998. This project represents much of the work and thoughts of Ron and others at The Center for Universal Design on what features and design elements should be incorporated in a universally designed home. A detailed drawing was prepared to illustrate the many universal features one might find in the home (Figure 1). The Next Generation Universal Home is a concept design of ideal and desired universal design features in single-family housing. Many of these features presently exist, yet it is unlikely to find all of them included in one home. This home design has not yet been built.

Entrances and Interior Passages. The home design is presented in

FIGURE 1. First and Second Floor Overview of The Next Generation Universal Home

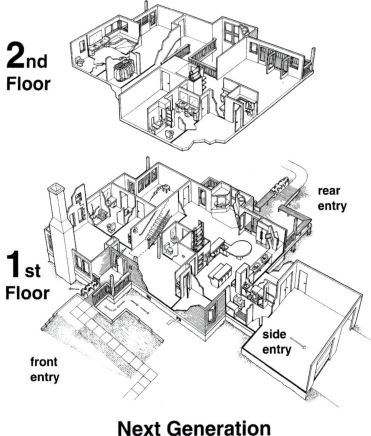

2nd Floor

1st Floor

rear entry

side entry

front entry

Next Generation Universal Home

two floors (Figure 2); how people use the upper floor will be addressed later in this paper. The house is designed so that all three entrances are usable–the front entrance, the entrance at the garage, and the entrance from the rear deck. At the main entrance, a feature called the "earth berm and bridge" is used to make up the difference in elevation between the house and street level (Figure 3). This feature is designed using an attractive retaining wall and landscaping. Soil is

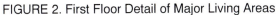

FIGURE 2. First Floor Detail of Major Living Areas

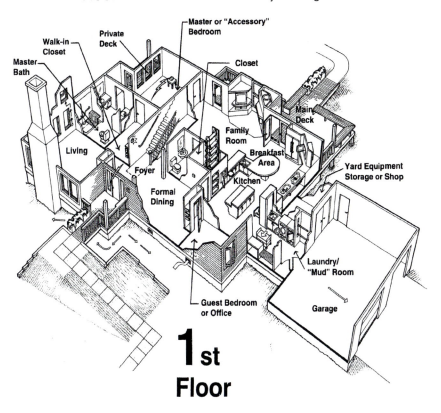

pushed up to the front of the house at the foundation. A bridge spans the gap to the gently sloping sidewalk. Ventilation and drainage are provided for. At the front entrance, a planter replaces one side of the handrails to protect someone from dropping off.

Other features at the main entrance include a package shelf for resting personal objects when unlocking and opening the door. Covering provides protection from the rain and wind. A doorbell and intercom at the latch side of the door provide communication with the homeowner. In this design, sidelights on both sides of the door provide visual contact from the inside with guests as they arrive. The house number is large and high contrast to be easily seen from the street. Focused lighting at the door is another security and convenience feature. Lever-style hardware makes opening the door easy for

FIGURE 3. Front Entry Showing Level Bridge to Door, Plant Stand to Prevent Drop Off, Convenient Package Shelf, Sidelight for Viewing Visitors, and Doorbell Intercom System

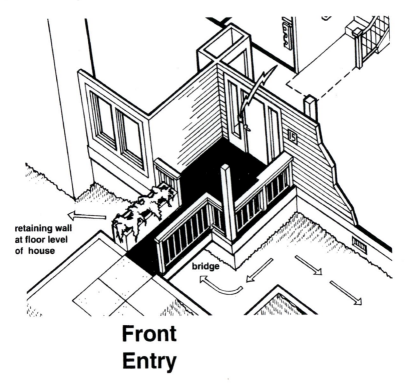

Front Entry

people with limited hand function or whose hands are full. Some examples of universal features for entrances are shown in Table 1.

Entrance and exit doors are all 36 inches wide. Inside the home, interior passage and closet doors provide at least a 32-inch clear opening. This allows easy maneuvering for people who use mobility aids, for moving furniture, or for two people passing in the hall. The same floor level throughout the first floor is a design element that can be appreciated by everyone. Home controls, such as the thermostat, should be easily reached by short and tall people, with visible and easily understood control functions. Some universal interior features are shown in Table 2.

Kitchen. In the kitchen, multiple work surfaces at different heights provide standing and seated users, as well as tall and short people,

TABLE 1. Entrances

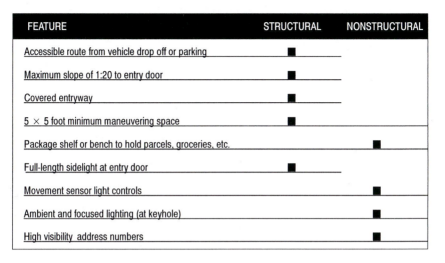

FEATURE	STRUCTURAL	NONSTRUCTURAL
Accessible route from vehicle drop off or parking	■	
Maximum slope of 1:20 to entry door	■	
Covered entryway	■	
5 × 5 foot minimum maneuvering space	■	
Package shelf or bench to hold parcels, groceries, etc.		■
Full-length sidelight at entry door	■	
Movement sensor light controls		■
Ambient and focused lighting (at keyhole)		■
High visibility address numbers		■

comfortable workspaces (Figure 4). Contrasting counter edges help locate the edge of the counter and can be used to surround the sink basin. All cabinet hardware features open loop handles to minimize fine finger manipulation. In this design, the primary sink and cooktop are located in an electrically operated, adjustable height counter. This is still an expensive feature that can be replaced by a manually adjustable counter. Knee space is provided under the sink and cooktop to ease use by seated users. Adjacent to the primary sink is a raised dishwasher to minimize bending to load and unload. Full extension drawers provide deep storage with easy access for all users.

The kitchen island has a lower work surface with open knee space. Note the peninsula table that can be used for dining as well as a lowered work surface. The secondary, or bar, sink has retractable doors that reveal open knee space. The faucet at this sink is mounted at the side of the basin to minimize reach distance. Two ovens are provided; one is a conventional oven mounted with the oven rack at the same height as the adjacent work surface, allowing the user to easily slide hot food across. The microwave oven is also set at counter height with a front shelf so hot or heavy dishes can be easily slid to a safe resting area. The refrigerator is a side-by-side design with refrigeration and freezer units adjacent to each other providing easy access to both. The unit is elevated to provide more storage space within com-

TABLE 2. General Interior

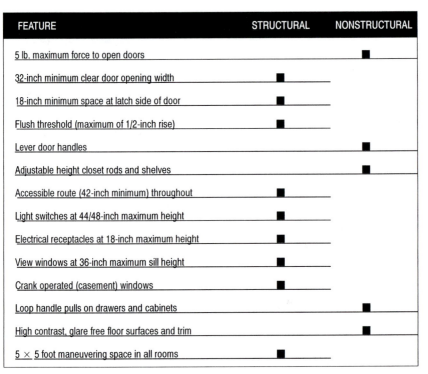

FEATURE	STRUCTURAL	NONSTRUCTURAL
5 lb. maximum force to open doors		■
32-inch minimum clear door opening width	■	
18-inch minimum space at latch side of door	■	
Flush threshold (maximum of 1/2-inch rise)	■	
Lever door handles		■
Adjustable height closet rods and shelves		■
Accessible route (42-inch minimum) throughout	■	
Light switches at 44/48-inch maximum height	■	
Electrical receptacles at 18-inch maximum height	■	
View windows at 36-inch maximum sill height	■	
Crank operated (casement) windows	■	
Loop handle pulls on drawers and cabinets		■
High contrast, glare free floor surfaces and trim		■
5 × 5 foot maneuvering space in all rooms	■	

fortable reach range. A final design feature is the moving shelf storage system that increases food storage within minimal space. This is a convenient feature for people who cannot reach high or deep. Table 3 shows some universal features in the kitchen.

Laundry. In the laundry area a rolling cart provides flexible storage and easy clothes handling (Figure 5). The bench is a place to rest while removing shoes or when waiting for clothes washing to finish. An adjustable height closet rod provides convenient hanging for people who are tall or short. The front loading washer and dryer reduce the need to reach far when placing or removing clothes. Controls are located at the front of the units. The wash basin is raised providing clear toe space. A laundry chute drops clothes from the second floor, reducing the need to carry clothes downstairs. In the garage, the floor slopes away from the house toward the vehicle door. Venting is provided to reduce build up of gas fumes.

FIGURE 4. Kitchen Showing Multiple and Adjustable Height Work Surfaces with Open Knee Space, Peninsula Table, Side-by-Side Refrigerator, Appliances at Convenient Heights, and Moving Shelf Storage System

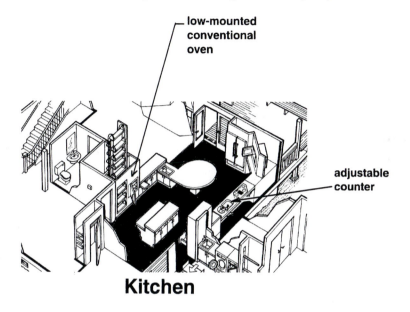

low-mounted conventional oven

adjustable counter

Kitchen

Master Bedroom and Bath. The master bathroom incorporates many universal design features (Figure 6). Dual lavatories, one low with open knee space and the second at conventional height with a base cabinet below, provide flexible use for the homeowner. A conceptual design is the multimode bathing fixture developed by Ron Mace. Three different bathing modes are provided in the same space–submerged in the water, seated on the bench, and standing. This design embodies universal design principles, such as flexible use. Grab bars can be included during construction, or added later on if reinforcement (wall blocking) is provided. Clear floor space–a 5-foot turning radius–provides adequate room for someone who uses a wheelchair to safely transfer to the toilet. Universal features in bathrooms are shown in Table 4.

Living Areas and Stairs. A clear story, or upper window, that can be operated with a motorized or manual opener has been placed in the living room. The lower window is operated with a simple to use crank handle. The family room features a raised hearth so that people who

TABLE 3. Kitchens

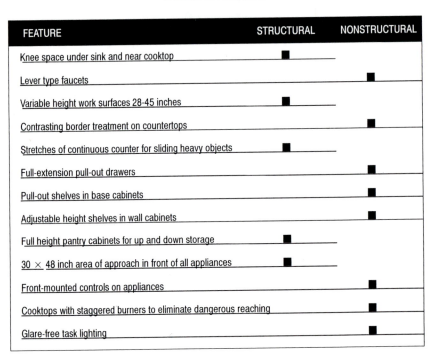

FEATURE	STRUCTURAL	NONSTRUCTURAL
Knee space under sink and near cooktop	■	
Lever type faucets		■
Variable height work surfaces 28-45 inches	■	
Contrasting border treatment on countertops		■
Stretches of continuous counter for sliding heavy objects	■	
Full-extension pull-out drawers		■
Pull-out shelves in base cabinets		■
Adjustable height shelves in wall cabinets		■
Full height pantry cabinets for up and down storage	■	
30 × 48 inch area of approach in front of all appliances	■	
Front-mounted controls on appliances		■
Cooktops with staggered burners to eliminate dangerous reaching		■
Glare-free task lighting		■

are seated can reach the fireplace. Controls at the TV/entertainment area are located low for use by seated users and children. At the central stairway, a smoke alarm incorporates an audible and visible alert signal for people who cannot see the alarm or who cannot hear it. The stairs to the second floor have been built wide enough to allow later installation of a stair lift. A nearby electrical outlet is needed to provide power for a lift or for safety lighting. Handrails extend at the top and bottom of the stairs for added support by some users. Contrasting treads and risers can aid people with low vision or when the lighting is dim. Another solution to provide access to the second floor, shown adjacent to the front powder room, are stacked closets where an interior elevator can later be added.

Second Floor. On the second floor, common design elements are again found in the two bathrooms (Figure 7). This includes knee space beneath the sink, dual or adjustable height sinks, adequate turning space at the toilet for people with mobility aids, and mirrors that

FIGURE 5. Features in Laundry Room Include Rolling Storage Cart, Resting or Folding Bench, Adjustable Height Clothes Rod, Front-Loading Appliances, and Raised Wash Basin

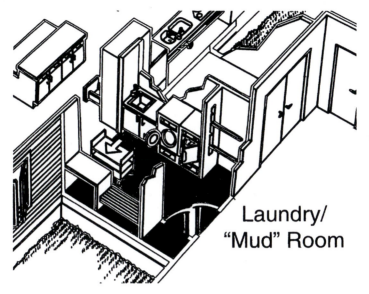

extend down to the lavatory. The front bathroom incorporates a conventional tub with an integral fold down seat with an adjustable height showerhead. Controls set to the outside of the tub allow easier and safer bathing. Pull-out storage is used again for easier access to linens and other bathing supplies. The rear upstairs bathroom features a wet area shower. In this design, modified from Japanese bathing, many options are provided. These include full standing, seated, or roll-in shower, and a soaking tub. One final feature upstairs is a motorized carousel to bring clothes to the front of the closet for easy access.

CONCLUSION

For universal design to become common practice rather than the exceptional, it must become more widely accepted as a beneficial concept for everyone. Universal design needs to be adopted by the housing industry as part of common practice in producing consumer products and new construction. Although it is growing in understand-

FIGURE 6. The Master Bath Features Dual Lavatories at Different Heights with Open Knee Space Below, a Multi-Mode Bathing Fixture, and Clear Floor Space for Wheelchair Users or to Allow Assistance by a Care provider

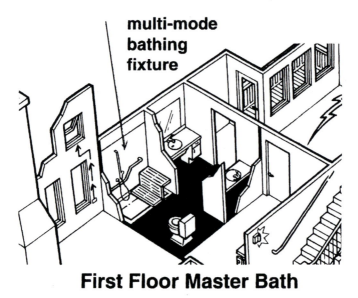

multi-mode bathing fixture

First Floor Master Bath

ing and acceptance, the industries that produce the built environment are large and complex and systemic change takes time and many kinds of efforts and supports.

The impact of recent civil rights legislation and a growing aging population has increased consciousness among designers, building owners, and manufacturers about the rights of people with a range of disabilities and the requirements for more accessible public and private places (Welch, 1995). By heightening the awareness of designers to a previously marginalized group of users, inclusive design values are more likely to be included in design discourse (Welch, 1995). People are disabled by situations and attitudes; a designer can meet the letter of the law, follow the details of the standards, and still not create an enabling environment.

Work thus far indicates that the need and market for universal design cannot be confirmed through conventional market analyses because it is not popular or pleasant to identify as having needs be-

TABLE 4. Bathrooms

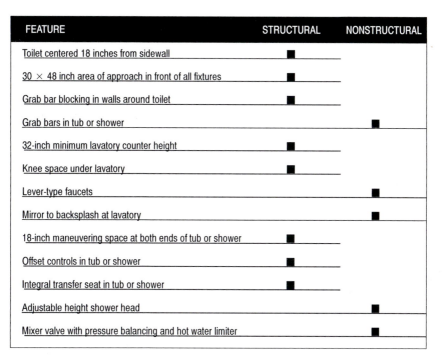

FEATURE	STRUCTURAL	NONSTRUCTURAL
Toilet centered 18 inches from sidewall	■	
30 × 48 inch area of approach in front of all fixtures	■	
Grab bar blocking in walls around toilet	■	
Grab bars in tub or shower		■
32-inch minimum lavatory counter height	■	
Knee space under lavatory	■	
Lever-type faucets		■
Mirror to backsplash at lavatory		■
18-inch maneuvering space at both ends of tub or shower	■	
Offset controls in tub or shower	■	
Integral transfer seat in tub or shower	■	
Adjustable height shower head		■
Mixer valve with pressure balancing and hot water limiter		■

cause of a disability or aging. Such needs are commonly regarded as special and outside the mainstream. Universal design attempts to address these needs within the mainstream. Strategies for pursuing universal design and measuring market response are needed, as are sensitive ways of communicating value and desirability of universal design without creating stigma.

The next steps are less about convincing people of the *need* for universal design (market forces, such as the baby boom generation, will in large part help drive demand for better design), but rather providing the *training and technical assistance* to show by example what universal design is and can be. This may include demonstration projects, dissemination through mass media, case studies, and other forms of technical assistance to customers who have committed to universal design projects. The Next Generation Universal Home is only a sample of what lies ahead.

FIGURE 7. The Second Floor Bath Demonstrates Open Knee Space Under and Adjustable Height of the Lavatories, an Integral Fold Down Seat to a Conventional Tub, Off-Set Faucet Controls, and Pull Out for Storage for Easier Access

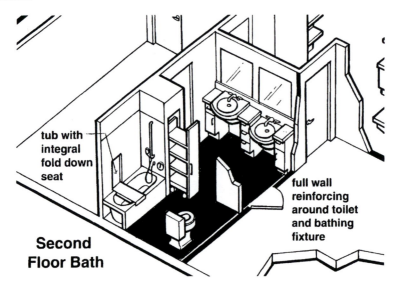

tub with integral fold down seat

full wall reinforcing around toilet and bathing fixture

Second Floor Bath

REFERENCES

Bednar, M. (1977). *Barrier Free Environments*. Stroudsburg, PA: Dowden Hutchinson, and Ross.

Mace, R. L., Hardie, G. J., & Place, J. P. (1991). Accessible Environments: Toward Universal Design. In Preiser, W. E., Vischer, J. C., & White, E. T. (Eds.), *Innovation by Design*. New York: Van Nostrand Reinhold.

Sanford, J. A., Story, M. F., and Ringholz, D. Consumer Participation to Inform Universal Design, *Technology and Disability* (in press).

Welch, P. (1995). *Strategies for teaching universal design*. Adaptive Environments, Boston, MA.

The Role of Occupational Therapists in Home Modification Programs at an Area Agency on Aging

Susan I. Klein, BSW, MA
Lois Rosage, MS, OTL/R
Geraldine Shaw, OTL/R

SUMMARY. The Housing Department of the Philadelphia Corporation for Aging (PCA) has administered home repair and modification programs for seniors since 1980. PCA now provides services to 1500 people annually through six programs. Currently funded at approximately four million dollars per year, PCA's Housing Department is the largest in any Area Agency on Aging.

In all these programs, PCA contracts with Occupational Therapist Consultants to assist the consumers and the programs to develop the most useful and appropriate modifications. In one program, serving Philadelphians of all ages, PCA has recently initiated a follow-up inspection by the therapist. These inspections are not only of benefit to the particular consumer, but also yield useful information on construction specifications and on the modification process. *[Article copies available for a fee from The Haworth Document Delivery Service: 1-800-342-9678. E-mail address: getinfo@ haworthpressinc.com <Website: http://www.haworthpressinc.com>]*

KEYWORDS. Home modifications, environmental assessments, community programs, aging in place, interdisciplinary teams

Susan I. Klein is Director of Housing, Philadelphia Corporation for Aging, 642 North Broad Street, Philadelphia, PA 19130-3409. Lois Rosage and Geraldine Shaw are Occupational Therapist Consultants who provide evaluations for the housing programs at the Philadelphia Corporation for Aging.

[Haworth co-indexing entry note]: "The Role of Occupational Therapists in Home Modification Programs at an Area Agency on Aging." Klein, Susan I., Lois Rosage, and Geraldine Shaw. Co-published simultaneously in *Physical & Occupational Therapy in Geriatrics* (The Haworth Press, Inc.) Vol. 16, No. 3/4, 1999, pp. 19-37; and: *Aging in Place: Designing, Adapting, and Enhancing the Home Environment* (ed: Ellen D. Taira, and Jodi L. Carlson) The Haworth Press, Inc., 1999, pp. 19-37. Single or multiple copies of this article are available for a fee from The Haworth Document Delivery Service [1-800-342-9678, 9:00 a.m. - 5:00 p.m. (EST). E-mail address: getinfo@haworthpressinc.com].

There are a limited number of programs across the country that provide home modifications and most of these are small (National Resource and Policy Center on Housing and Long Term Care, 1991; Pynoos, 1992). Agencies are usually isolated from one another and therefore, use a variety of assessment tools, assessors, procedures and service criteria to determine the modifications to be made (Pynoos, Liebig, Overton & Calvert, 1997; Wilner, 1997).

Some assessments are check lists focused on safety issues. These can be valuable peer-to-peer tools to assist consumers in rethinking their environment. Other assessments are professionally administered. Nevertheless, having a professional tell a consumer what they should do doesn't insure the item will be obtained, installed or used. There can be a wide gap between a professional assessing a need and the successful use of a modification by an older consumer (Gitlin & Schemm, 1996; Gitlin, 1998a).

The collaborative process among the assessors, the family and the consumer is very important (R. J. Ohta & B. M. Ohta, 1997; Gitlin, Corcoran, & Leimiller-Eckhart, 1995). Yet, an effective assessment is only the beginning of the process. After deciding what should be done, there are few construction standards for residential retrofitting. As Dr. Sanford and colleagues (1997) discussed, most national accessibility standards are for commercial properties and are usually based on the needs of younger people with disabilities and not on the needs of seniors.

There is some information available about factors which predict home modification implementation in older adults. Gosselin, Robitaille, Trichey, and Maltais (1993) studied 255 subjects who were offered free home modifications; 69% of the subjects agreed to one or more home modifications. Gosselin et al. (1993) found that low income status, good housing conditions, no difficulty managing budget, and awareness of the need for home modifications predicted implementation.

A review of the literature does not yield a body of work that describes in very practical terms the role of the occupational therapist in home modification programs for the elderly. Most work has been done in the area of assistive technology rather than in home modifications. From a pragmatic perspective, programs need to know the minimal professional involvement that ensures quality as well as cost effectiveness. Testing of different program designs needs to be explored (Steinfeld & Shea, 1993; Gitlin, 1998b).

Although home modification programs continue to need evaluation and development of guidelines, there are many areas of the country with little or no assistance in home modifications for seniors. For professionals and consumers who are interested in bringing this issue to their community, resources such as *A Blueprint for Action: A Resource for Promoting Home Modifications* (Home Modification Action Coalition, 1997) and the Home Modification Action Project[1] are valuable supports.

This paper describes home modification programs in an Area Agency on Aging and the use of Occupational Therapists to assess consumers and their environment.

HOW THE HOUSING PROGRAMS STARTED

Philadelphia Corporation for Aging (PCA) is a nonprofit organization established in 1973 and designated by the Pennsylvania Department of Aging as the Area Agency on Aging (AAA) for Philadelphia County. PCA is one of 52 such agencies in Pennsylvania and one of 670 across the United States.[2] PCA's mission is to improve the quality of life of older Philadelphians and to assist them in achieving their maximum level of health, independence and productivity.

PCA's entry into the world of home repairs and modifications started with a matching grant from the U.S. Department of Housing and Urban Development (HUD) in 1980. PCA was one of 7 sites and the only AAA to be awarded a grant to do minor repairs for seniors. The HUD grant was for $50,000 and PCA received money from local foundations for the required financial match. With these grants, PCA hired full-time mechanics and the Senior Housing Assistance Repair Program (SHARP) was born.

While providing minor repairs in seniors' homes, we soon realized that the scope of service was too narrow and SHARP could provide additional help by also installing modifications. In 1983, SHARP received funding to install major modifications (e.g., first floor powder rooms, stair elevators) in five homes and minor modifications (e.g., grab bars, handheld showers) on a routine basis. With the inclusion of major modifications, it became apparent that PCA needed professional assistance in evaluating the needs of the consumers and the appropriateness of the modifications. This recognition provided the impetus for an association between the Housing Department of PCA and Occupational Therapy (OT) Consultants.

The SHARP program now serves 625 very low income older homeowners a year and is funded at 1.1 million dollars through the Pennsylvania Lottery and the City of Philadelphia's Community Development Block Grant. PCA has increased the amount and variety of services through five additional programs. These include a Medicaid waiver program for consumers over 60 years old, two of PCA's other long term care programs, a National Institutes of Aging research grant[3] and the Adaptive Modification Program (AMP) (see Appendix 1).

These programs differ in many ways: program purpose, population served, funding source, funding amount, scope of service, type of modifications, budget per home, and who approves the work. Nevertheless, the process of providing the modifications is similar in all of the programs. All include a social service component, an eligibility review, an evaluation by an OT, and construction inspections. The work recommended is reviewed, approved and ordered. After the modifications are installed by PCA's in-house and subcontracted staff, a post inspection by supervisory construction staff is conducted to insure completeness and quality. Recently, we initiated follow-up OT visits in the Adaptive Modification Program.

INITIAL OCCUPATIONAL THERAPY HOME EVALUATION

The role of the OT is to assess the person, the family, the home environment and the relationship of these factors within the context of the program's scope and purpose. The occupational therapist needs to fully understand the physical, social and environmental demands that are being placed on the individual. By encouraging the consumer to discuss their daily routine, the therapist can assist in recognizing and identifying the day-to-day difficulties. This collaborative process enables and empowers the consumer and the family to be the vital link in the modification process. Without this process, OTs could recommend items that may never be used.

It has been the experience of the OTs that conversational self-reporting by the consumer must be complemented by observation of performance of the activity. Comments from consumers such as "I do fine in the bathroom," or "You don't need to go out the back door, we don't use it often," are at most "introductions" to subjects that require thorough analysis. Both the trained therapist and the consumer gradually shape a clear understanding of the problems through the sharing of information, as it is only in this way that workable solutions can be defined and implemented.

The initial OT evaluation for the housing department at PCA has undergone several alterations over the years. Ongoing efforts to learn which modifications work for specific consumers have transformed the OT evaluation form into a more comprehensive document. Today we still consider the evaluation to be a work in progress (see Appendix 2).

The four main sections of the evaluation are (i) household composition and medical information, (ii) functional deficits resulting from medical problems, (iii) home assessment and (iv) problems with recommended modifications.

Household Composition and Medical Information

The form has space for information about all members of the consumer's household, including their ages, health conditions and whether they are available to assist the consumer. Knowledge of the household composition is required to better understand who will be using the modification and to identify those for whom the modification may be a barrier. For example, the installation of a raised toilet in the only bathroom in a home might not be a good solution if there are small children in the home.

Involving as many members of the household in defining problems as well as developing solutions increases the acceptance and usefulness of planned adaptations. Households are dynamic, interactive units that have an established history of dealing with the problems of their members, sometimes with varying degrees of effectiveness. Becoming aware of the consumer's household, its strengths, weaknesses, and dynamics, can be valuable information in anticipating resistance to the modifications and to instituting changes.

Medical information assists the therapist in considering the possible course of the disease or decline in function due to illness or injury. Since some PCA programs are available to a consumer only once, the rehabilitation prognosis is essential to the therapist in developing recommendations of what will best serve the consumer over time.

Functional Deficits Resulting from Medical Problems

Observations made by the therapist during a walk-through of the home with the consumer provide valuable insight into the consumer's abilities and limitations. It is at this time that the consumer is asked to perform or simulate tasks in each area of the home. Solutions should not be based on presumptions. As an example, the assumption that "all arthritics can benefit from a shower chair" might lead to a recommendation to install a shower chair for someone who prefers to get into the bath water, and therefore, this would be a useless intervention. Initial conversations open the door to experiential learning for both the OT and the consumer. The therapist learns from seeing a consumer reflexively reach for the sink and towel bar for support, listening to the creak of it pulling against the wall, as well as the shortness of breath caused by overexertion when attempting to stand. The consumer, doing the same activity, learns that the towel bar is a little loose and notices that the low toilet seat makes it very difficult to stand without pulling up on loose bathroom fixtures.

While perceiving oneself as able and competent is a cornerstone to health and wellness, it can be somewhat of a barrier to considering helpful adaptations in the home. Through experience, we have found that raising the concept of a "good" day compared to a "bad" day has been instrumental in helping the consumer consider changes that are initially perceived as not necessary or as "overdoing" it. While acknowledging the competency of the consumer as reflected by their "good" days, we can then consider the problems presented when illness flares without defining the individual as incompetent. Adaptations designed to maximize functioning throughout the oscillating levels of physical ability can then be perceived by the consumer as positive interventions.

Lists of problematic areas for the consumer and recommendations generated from the walk-through are discussed in detail with the individual. It is at this point that the occupational therapist provides training to the consumer and/or family in the use of modifications to insure maximal safety and greater independence.

Home Assessment

This section of the Occupational Therapy Evaluation Form compiles information about the structure of the house. Observation and data collection starts from the moment the OT gets out of the car. Walking up to the front door, s/he notes the number of steps, their condition, the location of railings and the condition of the walkways.

At the same time, a home is not just a collection of areas and sizes of doorways. Especially for older people, the house represents who they are, their values, their family and their history. The home has symbolic meaning as well as being a place of comfort. Nevertheless, we are still surprised when someone who needs a first floor powder room chooses not to have it installed because they would have to move their furniture. Sometimes we fail to understand precisely why someone does not accept this free help, but refusals happen regularly.

Finally, when all the problem areas have been discussed and the recommendations decided upon, it is explained to the consumer that if for any structural reasons the modifications cannot be installed, the occupational therapist will discuss alternate plans with PCA construction staff. By involving the individual in every step of the evaluation, we find that there is a better understanding of the proposed modifications and of the entire program.

As part of a 1997 consumer satisfaction survey, PCA sent a questionnaire to 140 recipients of AMP services. Of the 43 responses we received, 65% said that the occupational therapist recommended a modification or equipment that was different from or in addition to their original request. In all of these cases, the respondents found the additional modifications helpful. These responses indicate the importance of occupational therapy in consumer-driven programs.

COLLABORATION WITH CONSTRUCTION STAFF

Up to this point, we have emphasized the crucial role of communication between the OT and the consumer. Equally important to a quality outcome is a clear understanding between the OT and the construction professional of their very different worlds.

Philadelphia, the birthplace of our nation, is a city of row houses, narrow stairways, no front yards and multiple story dwellings often over 100 years old. This is the definition of an accessibility nightmare in the world of retrofitting. Standard solutions such as ramps, stairway elevators, exterior lifts and grab bars cannot always be installed due to architectural constraints.

The OT often believes that, if they can imagine it, PCA construction staff can make it happen. This assumption can lead to confusion and frustration between the therapist and the construction manager. The team needs more than a basic knowledge of construction if it is to create and implement adaptations in buildings with brick party walls, claw footed iron bathtubs, unheated "shed kitchens" or 12 marble steps leading to the front door.

For the programs that provide major modifications, whenever possible, a joint evaluation with PCA's construction manager takes place. During these assessments, a better understanding of each professional's expertise emerges and detailed construction issues become clarified.

City building codes also present a challenge to the therapist and mechanic. Few row homes can accommodate a ramp with the recommended slope, although the construction manager can identify the type and location for a vertical lift that will assist the consumer. Ramps and electric lifts need to be well thought out as a team, considering not only incline rate, but clear public walking space, availability of side alley ways, and the risk of vandalism. Stairway elevators also come in a variety of models with features that can promote safe function. On/off switches, shoulder harnesses and seat locks are as important as overall dimensions and warranties.

The OTs quickly learn that installing a toilet in the three feet by four feet space under the stairs is not a feasible solution to the need for first floor bathroom facilities. For example, retrofit bathrooms also need to be close to the main sewer line. Antiquated plumbing and electrical systems call for an understanding of installation needs for toilets and handheld showers.

Therapists must communicate as thoroughly with the mechanics as they do with every other person involved in the adaptation. When workmen gain a better knowledge of the true functional problem, they can create structural solutions that are far more efficient than the medically trained individual. Many discussions are needed before each team member reaches true appreciation of the essential role of the other.

FOLLOW UP

The Adaptive Modification Program (AMP) can spend up to $25,000 per property for modifications. As such, the modifications under this program can have a dramatic impact on people's lives. Nevertheless, it became clear that some consumers were not using their modifications safely. As a result, PCA has recently instituted routine follow-up visits by the OT for all consumers in AMP.

In general, the OTs find follow-up visits professionally very reward-ing. The visit allows them to see positive changes in many areas of the lives of consumers resulting from the installation of the modification. Consumers can now do activities that they could not previously do.

Some follow-up visits are difficult to arrange because the consumers are using their newly found freedom and are rarely at home. Other modifications create a positive ripple effect for the consumers and their family. Consumers have increased social interaction because they are more comfortable having people in their homes after the installation of first floor powder rooms. Families have painted the living rooms to match the new powder rooms and others have decorated them. The OTs have been very pleased with the modification outcomes.

One of the goals of the follow-up visit is quality assurance. PCA is learning about gaps in our understanding of the problems and break-downs in the communication process among the consumers, the OTs, and the building contractors. These problems became apparent when the OT observed grab bars and handheld showers poorly placed, thresholds that are difficult to negotiate, a bathroom that has not been used and roll-in showers with faucets installed at a height suitable only for a person who stands in the shower. While the program has succeeded in preventing repetition of these mistakes rather quickly, follow up continues to be an essential component of the learning process for all concerned.

Primarily, the Occupational Therapists are finding the need to "tweak" the installation by small changes and to provide education to improve on the safe utilization of adaptations. The critical lessons that we are learning are related to communication and implemention.

Not all consumers are totally satisfied with the modification and as a result they do not make use of it. Regardless of how much commu-nication is emphasized, the finished product is a reality that cannot always be fully anticipated. Sometimes the OT finds the consumer disappointed or not using the modification because his or her disap-pointment is founded on the realization that everything is not as it was before the loss in function. In spite of a long process and considerable expense, the consumer is still left with the frustration of having diffi-culty accomplishing something that was once effortless. When listen-ing to complaints about seemingly minor or inconsequential details, the therapist needs to validate the consumer's remaining anger.

Acceptance of improved function over total restoration begins at the first visit. All staff must avoid a salesman-like approach that promises perfection. Focusing on individual task achievement has been our best strategy. From the beginning of the modification process, the OT must be clear that together we are coming up with solutions that improve or prevent problems and that reduce the risk of further injury.

Some people have been slow or reluctant to utilize modifications. This is especially frustrating for the therapist when the modifications are extensive. Again, therapists must not underestimate the complexity of the individual's coping strategies, the comfort with the "known" despite its lack of effectiveness, the impact on family dynamics of the newly designed space and the time needed for adjustment to any major life change. It often takes several months for a consumer to move up to the newly accessible first floor from the cramped, limiting basement, which had been home for several years.

CASE EXAMPLE

Ms. M is a 69 year old African-American woman with a diagnosis of diabetes mellitus, end stage renal disease, hypertension, congestive heart failure, and bilateral below the knee amputations. Her doctor described her condition as chronic/stable, reported that her prognosis was fair and estimated that she would use the planned adaptations for more than two years. Ms. M lives alone in a 2 story row house that has 3 brick steps leading to the front door. She has occupied only the first floor since her amputations several years ago and did not have a first floor toilet at the time of referral. Her hospital bed is in the living room with a portable commode positioned for a "straight on" transfer. She is transported via Paratransit to dialysis 3 times a week and had been carried, in her wheelchair, up and down her 3 exterior steps to reach the van. Neighbors were her main source of support for cooking, cleaning and shopping.

As a result of the initial occupational therapy evaluation, the following problems were identified: access in and out of her home; access to toilet; access to bathing facilities; and access to the kitchen area for meal preparation. After extensive discussion with the consumer and the construction supervisor, the following modifications were planned:

1. Provide an electric exterior lift at the front entrance of the house.
2. Install an intercom system with electric door release at the front door with a remote station located beside the consumer's bed.

3. Construct a bathroom with a stall shower and transfer shower chair in the present dining room.
4. Lower the kitchen sink and open the area underneath to allow for wheelchair accessibility.

When the construction was completed, the OT went to the consumer's home to do an on-site follow-up visit. Ms. M was delighted with the changes to her home and expressed particular pleasure with her new bathroom. When asked by the OT to demonstrate how she was transferring to the toilet and shower chair, the consumer explained that she hadn't used the bathroom because she was more comfortable transferring from the bed to her commode. Further investigation revealed that both the toilet and shower chair required a lateral transfer and that a grab bar was necessary at both sites to insure a safe, independent maneuver. Also, it was found that a residential "handicapped height" toilet was still not high enough for an even lateral transfer from the wheelchair and a 4″ raised seat was added.

Use of the exterior lift was also less than optimal at the time of follow up. With consumer demonstration it became apparent that she was not as independent in its use as was initially anticipated. A small ramp had been installed inside the front door to smooth out the high threshold, but due to the narrow entranceway, the consumer could not propel her wheelchair up the short ramp without assistance. Grab bars were installed on both sides of the front door for added support so that Ms. M could negotiate the entranceway independently.

As a result of continued communication among all parties involved, the relatively minor changes implemented as a result of the follow-up visit increased the effectiveness of the modifications significantly. We have found that this situation is not uncommon. Consumers are often pleased with the modifications in their homes and are unaware of the full potential of these modifications to increase their independence. OT follow-up visits have taught us that many adaptations require slight adjustments and consumer training to reach their intended purpose of maximal function.

CONCLUSION

Although PCA has had a long history in providing modifications, the process is always one of learning how to improve the quality of the product for the consumer. The modification process must be individualized to consider the physical, mental, and social needs of the consumer in relation to their environment. Routine occupational therapy follow-up visits are providing an excellent mechanism to increase quality assurance.

NOTES

1. Home Modification Action Project, funded by the Archstone Foundation, University of Southern California, Andrus Gerontology Center.

2. To find the name of your local agency, contact the Eldercare Locator, a service of the National Association of Area Agencies on Aging, at 1-800-677-1116.

3. Through a contract with Thomas Jefferson University, College of Heath Professions, Community and Homecare Research Division, Laura N. Gitlin, PhD, Principal Investigator, Philadelphia REACH study, funded by the National Institute on Aging, 5UO1 AG13265.

REFERENCES

Gitlin, L. (1998a). From hospital to home, individual variations in experience with assistive devices among older adults. In D. B. Gray, L. Quatrano & M. L. Lieberman (Eds.), *Designing and using assistive technology: The human perspective*, (pp. 117-135). Baltimore: Paul H. Brookes Publishing Co.

Gitlin, L. (1998b). Testing home modifications interventions: Issues of theory, measurement, design, and implementation. In R. Schulz, G. Maddox, & M. P. Lawton (Eds.), Focus on interventions research with older adults. *Annual Review of Gerontology and Geriatrics, 18*, 190-246.

Gitlin, L., Corcoran M., & Leimiller-Eckhart, S. (1995). Understanding the family perspective: An ethnographic framework. *The American Journal of Occupational Therapy, 49*(8) 802-809.

Gitlin, L. & Schemm, R. (April 1996). Maximizing assistive device use among older adults. *Team Rehab*, 25-28.

Gosselin, C., Robitalle, Y., Trickey, F., & Maltais, D. (1993). Factors predicting the implementation of home modifications among eldery people with loss of independence. *Physical & Occupational Therapy in Geriatrics, 12*, 15-27.

Home Modification Action Coalition. (1997). *A blueprint for action: A resource for promoting home modifications*. Available from The Center for Universal Design, North Carolina State University, Box 8613, Raleigh, NC 27695-8613. (http://www2.ncsu.edu/nscu/design/cud).

National Resource and Policy Center on Housing and Long Term Care. (1991). *National directory of home modifications/repair programs*. Los Angeles: Andrus Gerontology Center.

Ohta, R. J. & Ohta, B. M. (1997). The elderly consumer's decision to accept or reject home adaptations: Issues and perspectives. In S. Lanspery & J. Hyde (Eds.), *Staying put: Adapting the places instead of the people* (pp. 79-89). Amityville, New York: Baywood Publishing Company.

Pynoos, J. (1992). Strategies for home modification and repair. *Generations, 16*(2), 21-26.

Pynoos, J., Liebig, P., Overton, J. & Calvert, E. (1997). The delivery of home modification and repair services. In S. Lanspery & J. Hyde (Eds.), *Staying put: Adapting the places instead of the people* (pp. 171-191). Amityville, New York: Baywood Publishing Company.

Sanford, J. A., Story, M. F. & Jones, M. L. (1997). An analysis of the effects of ramp slope on people with mobility impairments. *Assistive Technology, 9*(1), 22-33.

Steinfeld, E. & Shea, S. (1993). Enabling home environments: Identifying barriers to independence. *Technology and Disability, 2*(4), 69-79.

Wilner, M. (1997). Report of the first national invitational conference on home modification. In S. Lanspery & J. Hyde (Eds.), *Staying put: Adapting the places instead of the people* (pp. 263-272). Amityville, New York: Baywood Publishing Company.

APPENDIX 1

PHILADELPHIA CORPORATION FOR AGING
642 North Broad Street
Philadelphia, PA 19130-3409
Fiscal Year 1998

HOUSING DEPARTMENT

	SHARP	CAREGIVERS	LTC OPTIONS	AMP	WAIVER	REACH
Full Name	Senior Housing Assistance Repair Program	Family Caregivers' Support Program	Options Care Management Program	Adaptive Modification Program	Medicaid Waiver Services	Resources for Enhancing Alzheimer's Caregiver Health
Date Started	1980	1988	1989	1989	1996	1996
Purpose of Program	Provide minor repairs and adaptations the senior can no longer do for him/herself	Provide adaptations to assist the family caregiver in the process of caregiving	Maintain people in need of personal care (some who are nursing home eligible) in their own homes	Increase independence of persons with disabilities	Maintain nursing home eligible people in their own homes	To test whether environmental skill building and modifications support family caregiving
Funding Institutes Source	PA Lottery and Community Development Block Grant (CDBG)	PA General Funds	PA Aging Block Grant Funds	Community Development Block Grant (HUD)	PA Dept of Welfare (Medicaid)	National of Health National Institute on Aging National Institute of Nursing Research

APPENDIX (continued)

	SHARP	CAREGIVERS	LTC OPTIONS	AMP	WAIVER	REACH
FY 98 Funding	Lottery: $760,000 CDBG: $350,000	$96,484	$431,285	$2,000,000	$337,447	$60,800
FY 98 Production	625 homes	173 homes	377 homes	164 homes	344 homes	35 families received home modification interventions
Population Served	Elderly homeowners only	Caregivers of elderly family members	Seniors needing personal care and nursing home eligible people 18 years old and older	People of any age with permanent physical disabilities	Nursing home eligible persons 60 and older	Family caregivers of people with dementia
Types of Work	Primarily minor repairs and adaptations	Modifications and assistive devices only	Major and minor repairs and adaptations	Modifications only	Major and minor repairs, adaptations and appliances	Home modifications
Examples of Typical Work	Doors, locks, faucets, basement steps, smoke alarms, occupational therapy evaluations, bath tub adaptations, grab bars and railings	Bathroom modifications, railings, assistive devices	Major repairs such as roofs, electrical and plumbing, bathroom adaptations, railings, intercoms and first floor powder rooms	Stairglides, exterior wheelchair lifts, first floor bathrooms, ramps, kitchens, laundries and hard-wired smoke alarms	Major repairs, minor repairs, bathroom adaptations, railings, intercoms, first floor powder rooms and stairglides	Bathroom adaptations, lighting, activities devices, reorganization of items in the environment, safety proofing home, etc.
Client Eligibility	• over 60 • section 8 low income • owner/occupant • Philadelphia property • structurally sound	Participants in FCSP who have not exhausted the $2,000 modification allotment	Participants in Options Program with priority determined by Care Managers	• Philadelphia resident • Permanent physical disability • Section 8 moderate income • Could benefit from modifications	Participants in Waiver Program with priority determined by Care Managers	Participants must meet program criteria and be placed in the treatment group. Care receivers must show signs of dementia and be living with their family caregiver.
How to Apply	Call PCA's Housing Dept. 215-765-9000 Ext. 5222	Through PCA's Long Term Care Access Dept. 215-765-6580	Through PCA's Long Term Care Access Dept. 215-765-6580	Call Housing Consortium for Disabled Individuals (HCDI) 215-895-5692	Through PCA's Long Term Care Access Dept. 215-765-6580	Community & Homecare Research Division, Thomas Jefferson University 215-503-2897

APPENDIX 2

PHILADELPHIA CORPORATION FOR AGING
HOUSING DEPARTMENT
OCCUPATIONAL THERAPY EVALUATION

———— AMP ———— Options (1or 2) ———— FCSP (—— Copay) ———— SHARP———— Waiver

Enrollment/Request Date: ———————————————— Evaluation Date: ————————————

1. **DEMOGRAPHIC INFORMATION:**

Client: ———————————————————— Phone: ———————————— ZIP: ——

Address: ———————————————————— PCG: ————————————————

Case Manager: ———————————————— CM Phone:————————————————

Anticipated Problems serving this household: ——————————————————————————

Client's subjective housing needs: ————————————————————————————

2. **HOUSEHOLD COMPOSITION & MEDICAL INFORMATION:**

	Age	Relate	Ht/Wt	Art	DM	CVA	COPD	CHF	CAD	SDAT	HTN	Other
Client												

Assistance Available: ————————————————————————————————

3. **FUNCTIONAL DEFICITS RESULTING FROM MEDICAL PROBLEMS:**

SENSORY Does the client have:	No	Yes	Yes, but compensates	Comment
Vision loss (can't see steps, can't see small print or numbers, etc.)				
Hearing loss (can't hear doorbell, telephone, smoke alarm, etc.)				
Olfaction loss (can't smell if food is rotting, smoke and/or fire)				

APPENDIX 2 (continued)

PHYSICAL/ACTIVITY Can the client . . .	No	Yes	Yes, but with difficulty	Comment
Grasp (doorknobs, grab bars, handles on cabinets, etc.)				
Reach (into cabinets, to open door from w/c, etc.)				
Bend (to get into tub, pick up items, or access low cabinets, etc.)				
Lift (commode bucket, laundry basket, food tray, etc.)				

PHYSICAL/TRANSFERS What type of transfer does the client perform?	No	Yes	Level	Comment
Stand-Pivot-Sit				
Transfer board/slide				
Dependent lift				
Sit to Stand				

PHYSICAL/MOBILITY Method of mobility for:	Method	Device used	Comments
Interior of home			
Exterior of home			
Steps in and out of home			
Steps to 2nd floor/bsmt			

ADL and IADL Status What is the level of assistance for each?	I	Min A	Mod A	Max A	D	Comments
Feeding						
Hygiene						
Dressing						
Bathing						
Cooking						
Laundry						
Cleaning						
Shopping						

4. HOME ASSESSMENT:

Living Situation: —————— Story ———————— Condition: G   F   P

Front Entrance: _____

_____

Doorbell: ——— yes   ——— no   ——— broken

Can client answer door in a timely manner?   ——— yes   ——— no

Rear Entrance: ————————————————   Used for: _____

Bedroom: ———   1st floor   ———   2nd floor   ———   3rd floor

Bathroom: ———   old fashioned tub ———   OH shower   ———   vanity   ———   std toilet

            ———   modern tub   ———   HH shower   ———   sink   ———   H/C toilet

            ———   faucets: G P   ———   stall shower   ———   no sink

                                                      ———   faucets: G P

Kitchen: sink faucets: G P

             Comments on kitchen set-up/accessibility: _____

_____

Steps: ———   1st to 2nd   ———   2nd to 3rd

	straight or curved	wood banister	iron banister	second railing	number of steps	width of steps	condition
Interior							
Basement							

Location of Washer: ———   1st floor   ———   basement ———   none

Location of Dryer: ———   1st floor   ———   basement ———   none

Would client benefit from relocation of laundry facilities? ———   yes   ———   no

6. EQUIPMENT CURRENTLY USED:

     ———   Cane   ———   Wheelchair   ———   Bathroom Equipment

     ———   Walker   ———   Scooter   ———   Commode

     ———   Crutches   ———   Stairglide   ———   Hospital Bed

     ———   Other _____

APPENDIX 2 (continued)

7. INITIAL REQUEST:

_____ Bathroom Mods/Equipment	_____ 1st floor pwdr room	_____ wheelchair lift/ramp
_____ railings	_____ 1st floor full bath	_____ other (specify):
_____ intercom/door release	_____ stairglide	_____

8. PROBLEMS:

_____
_____
_____
_____
_____
_____
_____
_____
_____
_____
_____
_____
_____
_____
_____
_____
_____
_____
_____

ADDITIONAL COMMENTS: _____

_____
_____
_____
_____

9. RECOMMENDATIONS:

MEDICAL EQUIPMENT			WROUGHT IRON RAILINGS			
Item #	Price	Description	Location	L Ascend	R Ascend	Comments
			Party Wall			
			Int Step			
			Ext Front			
			Ext Rear			
			Basement			
			Other			

MODIFICATIONS & MECHANICAL EQUIPMENT:

_____

Occupational Therapist, Registered/Licensed

MODIFICATIONS & MECHANICAL EQUIPMENT:

_____

Occupational Therapist, Registered/Licensed

An *E* for *ADAAG*:
The Case for *ADA Accessibility Guidelines for the Elderly* Based on Three Studies of Toilet Transfer

Jon A. Sanford, MArch
Katharina Echt, PhD
Pascal Malassigné, MID, IDSA

SUMMARY. ADA accessibility guidelines are based primarily on the capabilities of young people, and as such may not compensate adequately for the range of comorbidities and secondary conditions that are common among older people with disabilities. This paper reviews findings from three studies of toilet transfer which suggest that ADA accessibility guidelines (ADAAG) for toilet and grab bar configurations do not meet the needs of older adults. The first study, a nationwide survey of people with mobility impairments, assessed difficulty with ADA-compliant and other toilet/grab bar configurations. The second, a laboratory study of grab bar use, evaluated the effectiveness of different grab bar configurations. Finally, the third study evaluated four new toilet designs

Jon A. Sanford and Katharina Echt are affiliated with the Rehab R&D Center, VAMC Atlanta, Decatur, GA. Pascal Malassigné is affiliated with VAMC Milwaukee, Milwaukee, WI.

The comparison of grab bar configurations was funded by the Department of Veterans Affairs, Rehabilitation Research and Development Service, Washington, DC, Project #E629-RA. The evaluation of toilet prototypes was funded by the Department of Veterans Affairs, Rehabilitation Research and Development Service, Washington, DC, Project #E666-RC. The national survey was funded by the Access Board, Washington, DC, Contract #QA930020.

[Haworth co-indexing entry note]: "An *E* for *ADAAG*: The Case for *ADA Accessibility Guidelines for the Elderly* Based on Three Studies of Toilet Transfer." Sanford, Jon A., Katharina Echt, and Pascal Malassigné. Co-published simultaneously in *Physical & Occupational Therapy in Geriatrics* (The Haworth Press, Inc.) Vol. 16, No. 3/4, 1999, pp. 39-58; and: *Aging in Place: Designing, Adapting, and Enhancing the Home Environment* (ed: Ellen D. Taira, and Jodi L. Carlson) The Haworth Press, Inc., 1999, pp. 39-58. Single or multiple copies of this article are available for a fee from The Haworth Document Delivery Service [1-800-342-9678, 9:00 a.m. - 5:00 p.m. (EST). E-mail address: getinfo@haworthpressinc.com].

39

with built-in handholds to facilitate transfer. Collectively, these studies indicate that there is a need for alternative ADA Accessibility Guidelines for the Elderly (ADAAGE). *[Article copies available for a fee from The Haworth Document Delivery Service: 1-800-342-9678. E-mail address: getinfo@ haworthpressinc.com <Website: http://www.haworthpressinc.com>]*

KEYWORDS. Toileting, bathing, transfer, accessibility, ADA, accessible/ universal design, aging in place, home modifications, independence, safety

BACKGROUND

Although the Americans with Disabilities Act Accessibility Guidelines (ADAAG) were initially issued in 1991, many of the guidelines were based on design standards for people with disabilities that were developed almost two decades ago. In the time since the development of these early standards, the demographics of the population of people with disabilities have changed dramatically. People are growing older and a larger number of individuals are living longer with disabilities (Bureau of the Census, 1983; 1992; Chirikos, 1986; Colvez & Blanchet, 1981; Jones & Sanford, 1996; Kunkel & Applebaum, 1992; LaPlante, Hendershot, & Moss; 1992; Zola, 1993). As a result, individuals' functional abilities may not be served by existing design guidelines. In fact, a number of researchers, including Czaja (1984), Faletti (1984), Sanford and Megrew (1995), and Steinfeld and Shea (1993), have argued that accessibility standards, based primarily on the capabilities of young people, may not compensate adequately for the range of comorbidities and secondary conditions that are common among older people with disabilities. As a consequence, adhering to accessibility codes in buildings used primarily by older people (e.g., senior centers and independent living facilities) or using codes as guidelines for home modifications when they are not specifically required by law, may do more to promote dependence among older people than to ameliorate it (Sanford & Megrew, 1995). This suggests that alternative guidelines based on the needs and capabilities of elderly individuals should be established.

The need to establish alternative ADA Accessibility Guidelines for the Elderly (ADAAGE) is based on three hypotheses:

H1. *Due to the aging of the population, the demographics of disability are changing such that traditional stereotypes of people with disabilities are no longer valid.*

H2. *Older people with disabilities have different functional abilities and therefore use the environment in different ways than people who fit the traditional stereotypes of disability.*

H3. *The lack of congruence between how older people use the environment and how ADAAG requires the environment to be designed creates demands that can exceed the competence levels (Lawton, 1986) of many older individuals with disabilities (i.e., is difficult to use, compromises safety, and promotes dependence).*

One area of concern that exemplifies the need for alternative guidelines is the usability of the preferred ADA toilet/grab bar configuration. Because the loss of ability to toilet independently often results in an elderly individual's relocation from the community to a nursing home, guidelines that facilitate independent transfer are particularly important for this population. This paper will review findings from three studies of toilet transfer which suggest that ADA accessibility guidelines for toilet and grab bar configurations do not meet the needs of older people with disabilities. The first study, a nationwide survey of people with mobility impairments, described a large random sample of people with disabilities (H1); examined transfer preference and difficulty (H2); and assessed difficulty with ADA-compliant and other toilet/grab bar configurations (H3). The two other projects were laboratory studies that evaluated the effectiveness of different grab bar and toilet designs. Collectively, these studies indicate that the preferred ADA toilet and grab bar configuration is more difficult and less safe for older individuals to use than several alternative, non-compliant configurations (H3).

DESCRIPTION OF PROJECTS

Project 1. National Survey of People with Mobility Impairments

Purpose. This project was sponsored by the Access Board, the Federal agency responsible for promulgating the ADA accessibility guidelines, for the purpose of identifying where further research is needed regarding space requirements for toilets, alternative grab bar designs and configurations, and the usability of fixtures according to various configurations. In addition, recommendations for changes to ADAAG were to be developed, where possible.

Methodology. The survey was mailed to a nationwide sample of 3278 people with mobility impairments. The sample was randomly selected from people in a large commercial database who were identified as having a disability. Respondents were asked to provide information about their age, gender, type of disability, length of impairment, and mobility aids used, as well as about transfer position and use of four commonly-found grab bar configurations (see Figure 1). The four included (1) the preferred ADA configuration with grab bars mounted on the walls beside and behind a toilet; (2) the alternative ADA configuration with grab bars mounted on walls 3 feet apart on both sides of a toilet; (3) a one-piece grab bar that straddled a toilet with projections on both sides and a cross bar behind the toilet; and (4) swing-away grab bars mounted on the wall behind the toilet, extending out on both sides of the toilet and capable of pivoting up and out of the way.

Project 2. Evaluation of Grab Bar Configurations to Meet the Needs of Older People

Purpose. The purpose of this study was to determine whether different grab bar configurations accounted for differences in difficulty, safety, and independence in toileting among older adults and whether

FIGURE 1. Toilet/Grab Bar Configurations

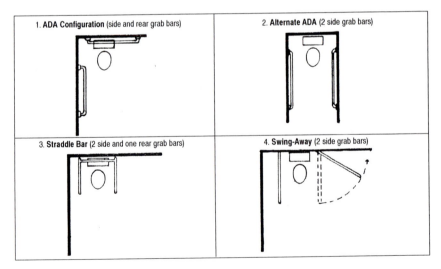

there were grab bar configurations that were more appropriate for older people than ADA code-compliant grab bars.

Methodology. A repeated measures design was used to test the effectiveness of the four grab bar configurations. One hundred and sixteen individuals 60+ years old participated in the study. Sixty-six (56.9%) of the participants were ambulatory[1] and 50 (43.1%) were nonambulatory. A full-scale, transportable mockup of a toilet room was fabricated. The mockup accommodated two videotape cameras to record the test trials, toilets mounted at 17 and 19 inches above the finished floor (representing the upper and lower limits in ADAAG), and four grab bar configurations each located at 33 and 36 inches (also the upper and lower height limits specified in ADAAG). The four grab bar configurations (see Figure 2) included (1) a configuration that complied with ADAAG; (2) a configuration that had a short bar beside the toilet and an ADA-compliant bar behind the toilet (often used

FIGURE 2. Grab Bar Configurations Tested

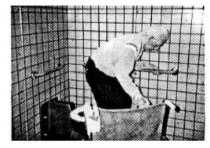

Preferred ADA configuration

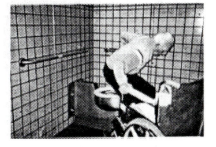

Configuration with short side bar

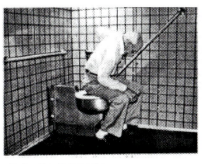

Configuration with diagonal bar

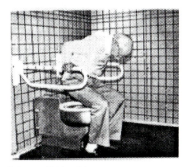

Swing-away Linido grab bars

when a door located on the side wall just in front of a toilet precludes the use of a longer grab bar); (3) a configuration that was the same as number 2 above, but with an additional diagonal grab bar; and 4) a configuration that included a swing-away grab bar on either side of the toilet.

A pretrial interview was conducted to solicit demographic information, cognitive status, and medical history for each participant. The test trials consisted of having each participant approach and get on the toilet, stay seated for a few seconds, and get off the toilet. Each trial was videotaped to assess grab bar use. Post-trial interviews solicited respondents' self-reports of perceived safety and ease of use of the grab bars using a 5 point Likert scale (where 1 = very difficult/unsafe and 5 = very easy/safe). Following completion of all trials, participants were given photographs of each configuration and asked to rank order the configurations for safety, ease of use, and personal preference.

Project 3. Design of New Toilet Prototypes for Older Individuals

Purpose. The purpose of this project was to develop and evaluate the effectiveness of three new toilet prototypes. The prototypes were designed to replace existing raised toilet seats and included integral handles or handholds to foster safer and more independent toileting among older individuals with mobility impairments when used in conjunction with wall-mounted grab bars.

Methodology. The same repeated measures design described in Project 2 above was used to evaluate the effectiveness of the prototypes. Subjects included individuals over 60 years of age who were capable of independent toileting and who stood to transfer onto a toilet. Two of the prototypes included integral handholds that could assist individuals who used either standing or sliding transfers. One of these prototypes had a recessed grip on each side of the seat platform (see Figure 3a); the other had cut-out handles on each side of the seat platform (see Figure 3b). The third prototype had vertical handles on each side and perpendicular to the seat platform (see Figure 3c) to assist individuals who performed standing transfers only.

Full-scale mockups of the prototype designs as well as a standard accessible toilet were installed in the portable test unit described above. In addition, ADA compliant, wall-mounted side and rear grab bars were provided. The same testing protocol described in the previous project was also used in this project, including the pretrial background information, test trials, and post-trial debrief. The test trials

FIGURE 3. Toilet Prototypes

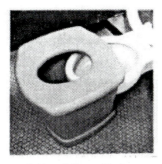

a. Prototype with Recessed Handles

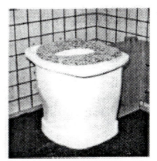

b. Prototype with Side Handles

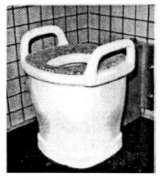

c. Prototype with Vertical Handles

consisted of asking each participant to approach and get on the toilet, stay seated for a few seconds, and get off. After each trial, participants were asked to evaluate their performance. The post-trial interviews consisted of a series of questions related to safety, ease or difficulty of use, and the helpfulness of the grab bars.

FINDINGS

H1. *Due to the aging of the population, the demographics of disability are changing such that traditional stereotypes of people with disabilities are no longer valid.*

A description of the sample of survey respondents provides important evidence that the population of people with disabilities is no longer comprised predominantly of young adults who use wheelchairs. The data portray a population of people aging into disability who sometimes use a wheelchair to compensate for limited strength and stamina, and who have difficulty standing up and sitting down, yet do not perform a sliding transfer directly between the wheelchair and toilet. Nonetheless, it is this latter type of transfer for which the preferred ADAAG toilet and grab bar configuration is intended.

From a random sample of almost 3300 people with disabilities, responses from 1193 individuals were included in the survey database. Almost two-thirds of the respondents (n = 785) were 55+ years of age, suggesting that older people represent a large percentage of the population of people with disabilities. Although it is possible that older individuals might have been more likely to respond to the survey, older respondents still accounted for almost one out of every four of the 3300 surveys distributed. Thus, even if the 785 older respondents represent all of the older individuals who received a survey (which is unlikely), the number of older respondents within the entire pool of participants would still have been substantial.

In general, older respondents had been impaired for a relatively short period of time. Over 60% of this group had been impaired for fewer than 10 years (see Table 1), which suggests that the majority of

TABLE 1. Type and Longevity of Impairment of Older Sample

Years with Impairment	N	% of Sample	Cumulative %
< 1	24	3.1	3.1
1-5	239	30.6	33.7
6-10	210	26.9	60.6
11-20	146	18.7	79.3
21-30	65	8.3	87.6
30 +	97	12.4	100.0
Total	781	100.0%	
Condition			
Hemiplegia	17	2.6	2.6
Poor Balance	364	55.4	58.0
Arthritis	165	25.1	83.1
Paraplegia	38	5.8	88.9
Quadriplegia	4	0.6	89.5
Amputation	69	10.5	100.0
Total	657	100.0%	

older respondents did not fit the traditional model of people aging with a disability. Rather, it portrays a large number of people who had aged into disability, having become impaired later in life.

Another indicator that the survey sample was different than the population of people with disabilities for whom ADAAG was intended was the type of conditions that people reported (Table 1). Whereas people with disabilities have traditionally been assumed to have conditions such as paraplegia, quadriplegia, and amputation, these conditions accounted for less than 20% of the sample. On the other hand, people with age-related conditions such as arthritis, poor balance, and hemiplegia (usually associated with stroke) accounted for more than 80% of the sample.

Finally, despite traditional stereotypes of people with disabilities as full-time users of wheelchairs, only 5.2% of the older sample used a wheelchair all of the time. In contrast, 47.4% did not use a wheelchair at all; and an additional 46.5% used wheelchairs some of the time, but typically used walking aids as well.

> H2. *Older people with disabilities have different functional abilities and therefore use the environment in different ways than people who fit the traditional stereotypes of disability.*

The preferred ADA grab bar configuration is designed to facilitate sliding transfers that are made directly from wheelchair to toilet, and back again. The side and rear grab configuration is based on the presumption that individuals who use wheelchairs will position themselves adjacent to the toilet (see Figure 1), reach across the toilet, and use the grab bars to pull themselves out of the wheelchair and slide onto the toilet. However, data from the survey revealed that more than 90% of the older respondents stood to transfer onto the toilet (see Table 2). This included all of the ambulatory individuals (n = 362) and 88.5% of the respondents who used wheelchairs (n = 355).

Therefore, it is not surprising that the front transfer position, which is most commonly used by ambulatory individuals with a standing

TABLE 2. Type of Transfer by Ambulatory Status

Ambulatory Status	N	Standing Transfer	Sliding Transfer
Ambulatory	362	362	0
Wheelchair user	401	355	46

transfer, was preferred by the largest percentage (33.6%) of wheel-chair users (see Table 3). Moreover, among wheelchair users who stood to transfer, the front transfer position had the lowest mean difficulty rating (mean = 2.85) on a 5-point Likert scale. Although the mean rating for front transfer was only slightly lower than the other configurations (see Table 4), it was significantly lower than the ratings for both parallel side transfers (mean = 3.30) and perpendicular transfers (mean = 3.31). Conversely, the front transfer was rated as the most difficult type of transfer (mean = 4.56) for respondents who used a direct sliding transfer between wheelchair and toilet, although the differences were not significant.

TABLE 3. Nonambulatory Respondents' Preference for Toilet Transfer Position

Transfer Type	n	% of wc users
a. parallel side transfer	65	9.3%
b. angled side transfer	50	14.9%
c. angled front transfer	60	17.9%
d. perpendicular transfer	48	14.3%
e. front transfer	113	33.6%
Total	336	100%

H3. *The lack of congruence between how older people use the environment and how ADAAG requires the environment to be designed creates demands that can exceed the competence levels of older individuals resulting in difficulty of use, compromised safety, and dependence.*

Data from all three projects indicate that older people had more difficulty using the preferred ADA toilet/grab bar configuration than a number of other configurations. Moreover, when alternative configurations were provided, older subjects more often used those that were better positioned and used mobility aids less often for supplemental support.

Difficulty and Safety. When survey respondents reported perceived difficulty of getting on and off a toilet by grab bar configuration, the preferred ADA configuration was the second most difficult of the four configurations[2] for two subgroups, semiambulatory (wheelchair users who stood to transfer) and ambulatory (used walking aids or no aid). Moreover, post hoc comparisons showed that the ADA configuration was significantly more difficult than the alternate ADA and straddle configurations for these two groups (see Table 5). Both the alternate ADA configuration and straddle configurations are intended to facilitate a standing, front transfer by enabling individuals to grasp the grab

TABLE 4. Effect of Transfer Type and Position on Difficulty Among Wheelchair Users

Transfer Type	N	Mean[a]	Standard Deviation	Sig. level	Significant Post Hoc Comparisons*
Standing Transfer					
a. Parallel Side	188	3.30	1.41	.004	d
b. Angled Side	187	3.25	1.40		
c. Angled Front	190	3.09	1.40		
d. Front Transfer	196	2.85	1.37		a, e
e. Perpendicular	192	3.31	1.32		e
Total	*953*	*3.16*	*1.39*		
Sliding Transfer					
a. Parallel Side	33	3.87	1.38	ns	
b. Angled Side	35	3.81	1.28		
c. Angled Front	34	4.10	1.19		
d. Front Transfer	33	4.56	0.82		
e. Perpendicular	35	3.99	1.17		
Total	*170*	*4.06*	*1.20*		

[a] Likert rating scale where 1 = very difficult and 5 = very easy
* p < .02

TABLE 5. Effect of Configuration on Difficulty by Ambulatory Status

Ambulatory Status	N	Mean	Standard Deviation	Sig.	Significant Post Hoc Comparisons*
Nonambulatory					
a. ADA Configuration	30	2.97	1.49	ns	
b. Alternate ADA	30	3.63	1.29		
c. Straddle	31	3.52	1.29		
d. Swing-away	30	3.30	1.19		
Total	*121*	*3.36*	*1.33*		
Semiambulatory					
a. ADA Configuration	199	2.64	1.14	.000	b, c
b. Alternate ADA	201	2.03	1.04		a, d
c. Straddle	193	2.04	1.10		a, d
d. Swing-away	180	2.71	1.43		b, c
Total	*773*	*2.35*	*1.22*		
Ambulatory					
a. ADA Configuration	280	2.33	1.05	.000	b, c
b. Alternate ADA	284	1.71	0.89		a, d
c. Straddle	258	1.83	1.06		a, d
d. Swing-away	233	2.50	1.42		b, c
Total	*1055*	*2.08*	*1.15*		

ADA Configuration	Alternate ADA	Straddle Bar	Swing-Away

*$p \leq .001$

bars on both sides of the toilet to pull themselves out of the wheelchair or off the toilet to a standing position, pivot, and sit down. Therefore, it is not surprising that these two were the least difficult for subjects who performed standing transfers. However, it should be noted that the alternative ADA configuration is permissible only in renovations where sufficient space is not available for the preferred configuration, irrespective of whether the users perform standing or sliding transfers.

Finally, although the preferred ADA configuration was the least difficult configuration for the nonambulatory group, differences in mean ratings between configurations were not significant. This suggests that even among older people who use a sliding transfer, the preferred ADA configuration is no less difficult than any of the others, including those intended for standing transfers.

Patterns of difficulty of grab bar use in the laboratory studies were similar to those described in the survey study. In addition, findings from the grab bar study indicate that there were grab bar configurations that were safer for, and more preferable to, older subjects than the preferred ADA configuration. In fact, the preferred configuration rated next to last in safety, ease, and preference by both nonambulatory and ambulatory participants in this study (Table 6). However, in contrast to the survey respondents who rated the swing-away grab bars as difficult to use, nonambulatory and ambulatory subjects who actually used these grab bars rated the configuration safest (54.8% and 45.8%, respectively) and easiest to use (58.5% and 46.6%, respectively). Although these ratings were significantly different for the nonambulatory group, there were no significant differences among ambulatory participants in ratings of safety or difficulty ratings between swing-away grab bars and a second non-ADA compliant configuration that included a diagonal bar. Moreover, whereas 31.6% of the

TABLE 6. Subjects' Self-Report of Grab Bar Use

Group	Ratings									
	Safest		Least Safe		Easiest		Most Difficult		Best	
	n	%	n	%	n	%	n	%	n	%
Nonambulatory										
ADA Configuration	6	14.3	6	17.1	5	12.2	7	19.4	7	16.7
Configuration w/ short side grab bar	2	4.8	16	45.7	2	4.9	18	50.0	2	4.8
Swing-away grab bars	23	54.8	7	20.0	24	58.5	5	13.9	26	61.9
Configuration w/ diagonal grab bar	11	26.2	6	17.1	10	24.4	6	16.7	7	16.7
Total	42	100.1	35	99.9	41	100.0	36	100.0	42	100.1
Chi-square	23.274		8.086		27.78		12.222		32.095	
p	≤.0001		.0443		≤.0001		.0067		≤.0001	
Ambulatory										
ADA Configuration	6	10.2	6	11.1	3	5.2	5	10.0	5	8.8
Configuration w/ short side grab bar	2	3.4	31	57.4	2	3.4	29	58.0	4	7.0
Swing-away grab bars	27	45.8	9	16.7	27	46.6	8	16.0	18	31.6
Configuration w/ diagonal grab bar	24	40.7	8	14.8	26	44.8	8	16.0	30	52.6
Total	59	100.1	54	100.0	58	100.0	50	100.0	57	100.0
Chi-square	32.186		30.593		39.793		29.52		31.772	
p	≤.0001		≤.0001		≤.0001		≤.0001		≤.0001	

ambulatory group rated the swing-away configuration as the best, 52.6% preferred the diagonal bar arrangement.

Finally, in the project that developed and evaluated three new toilet prototypes, the effectiveness of the prototypes was compared not only among each other, but to the preferred ADA configuration as well. Using self-report and observational data collection methods developed for the study of grab bar configurations, both types of data again indicated that there were toilet configurations better suited to the elderly population than the preferred ADA configuration.

In this study, almost 70% of the subjects reported that the ADA-compliant toilet and grab bar configuration was the most difficult to use, although a larger number felt that it was safer and better than the prototypes with recessed or side handles (Table 7). In contrast, 60% of the subjects rated the prototypes with vertical handles as the safest and 63.6% rated it as the best. These findings are not surprising, as the vertical handles were intended to ameliorate problems older people experience due to a lack of support below the grab bars and above the toilet seat to assist their transition from sit-to-stand positions.

Frequency of Use of Grab Bars and Mobility Aids. Grab bar use is an indicator of the appropriateness of the placement of the grab bar. Simply put, when grab bars are located within comfortable reach of an older individual, they provide a greater opportunity to be used than when they are not located within easy reach. Therefore, the more appropriately a grab bar is positioned for a specific transfer position, the more often it will be used.

In the grab bar study, frequency of grab bar use was determined by counting the number of ways in which each grab bar was used: (1) pulling oneself out of a wheelchair or off the toilet; (2) support

TABLE 7. Subjects' Self-Report of Toilet Prototype Use

	Toilet Type							
	ADA Configuration		Prototype w/ Recessed Handles		Prototype w/ Side Handles		Prototype w/ Vertical Handles	
	n	%	n	%	n	%	n	%
Safest	6	30.0	0	0	2	10.0	12	60.0
Most Difficult	11	68.8	1	6.3	2	12.5	3	18.8
Best	5	22.7	2	9.1	1	4.5	14	63.6

while standing; (3) stability while pivoting; and (4) assistance for lowering oneself onto the toilet or wheelchair. Thus, each grab bar could have been used a total of 928 times [4 types of uses × (116 trials getting on + 116 getting off)].

The swing-away grab bars were used significantly more often (p ≤ .0001) by both ambulatory and nonambulatory participants (see Table 8), accounting for 40% (551 out of 1371) of all grab bar uses and the highest percentage (59.4%) of all possible grab bar uses (see Table 9). In slight contrast to the self-report ratings, the preferred ADA configuration not only had the least number of uses of any of the four configurations, it was used only half as often as the swing-away grab bars to get on the toilet (n = 131 compared to 268) and less than half the number of times to get off (n = 121 compared to 283 uses). Similarly, the ADA configuration had the lowest ratio of actual grab bar use to possible grab bar use (27.2%) of the four configurations (see Table 9).

Another indicator of the effect of different grab bar configurations

TABLE 8. Frequency of Grab Bar Use by Configuration and Ambulatory Status

Group	Transfer On n (%)	Transfer Off n (%)	Total Uses (%)
Nonambulatory			
ADA Configuration	75 (17.1%)	65 (17.6%)	140 (17.3%)
Configuration w/ short side grab bar	91 (20.7%)	69 (18.7%)	160 (19.8%)
Swing-away grab bars	170 (38.6%)	156 (42.3%)	326 (40.3%)
Configuration w/ diagonal grab bar	104 (23.6%)	79 (21.1%)	183 (22.6%)
Total uses	440 (100%)	369 (100%)	809 (100%)
Chi-square	*47.473*	*59.867*	
p	*≤ .0001*	*≤.0001*	
Ambulatory			
ADA Configuration	56 (21.2%)	56 (18.8%)	112 (19.9%)
Configuration w/ short side grab bar	44 (16.7%)	53 (17.8%)	97 (17.3%)
Swing-away grab bars	98 (37.1%)	127 (42.7%)	225 (40.0%)
Configuration w/ diagonal grab bar	66 (25.0%)	62 (20.8%)	128 (22.8%)
Total uses	264 (100%)	298 (100%)	562 (100%)
Chi-square	*24.364*	*49.893*	
p	*≤.0001*	*≤.0001*	

was the frequency of use of wheeled mobility devices (wmds) to assist in transfer (see Table 10). Because subjects held onto whatever object they could reach most easily, mobility devices which could become unsteady, rather than grab bars, were used when the grab bars were improperly positioned. As a result, use of mobility devices was significantly higher than grab bar use in all configurations (p = .0021) except the configuration with swing-away grab bars, where the number of uses was significantly lower for transfer on (p = .005) and lower (although not significantly) for transfer off.

Similar results regarding use of wmds were found in the evaluation of toilet prototypes. Findings from this study (see Table 11) indicate that a significant increase in use of integral handles (p ≤ .0011) across prototypes was accompanied by a corresponding and significant decrease in the use of wmds (p ≤ .0001). Furthermore, data indicate that increased use of integral handles was accompanied by a concomitant

TABLE 9. Frequency of Use and Percentage of Possible Grab Bar Uses by Configuration

Configuration	Transfer On (N)	Transfer Off (N)	Total Number of Uses	Percentage of Possible Use (928)
ADA Configuration	131	121	252	27.2
Configuration w/short side grab bar	135	122	257	27.7
Swing-away grab bars	268	283	551	59.4
Configuration w/ diagonal grab bar	170	141	311	33.5
Total number of uses	704	667	1371	

TABLE 10. Frequency of Mobility Device Use in Transfer (Nonambulatory Subjects)

Configuration	Transfer On n (%)	Transfer Off n (%)	Total Uses
Configuration 1	152 (24.7%)	128 (22.6%)	280 (23.7%)
Configuration 2	189 (30.7%)	162 (28.6%)	351 (29.7%)
Configuration 3	122 (19.8%)	139 (24.6%)	261 (22.1%)
Configuration 4	152 (24.7%)	137 (24.2%)	289 (24.5%)
Total uses	615 (100%)	566 (100%)	1181 (100%)
Chi-square	*14.678*	*ns*	
p	*.0021*		

TABLE 11. Frequency of Device Use

	ADA Configuration	Prototype Rec. Handles	Prototype Side Handles	Prototype Vertical Handles	Total Uses	Chi-square *p-value*
Grab Bars	184	173	159	124	640	12.763 *.0052*
Integral Handles	---	39	54	78	171	13.579 *.0011*
Mobility Devices	108	92	78	69	347	29.897 *.0001*
Total uses	292	304	291	271	1158	ns
Chi-square *p-value*	19.781 *.0001*	89.891 *.0001*	62.412 *.0001*	19.27 *.0001*	290.834 *.0001*	

and significant decrease (p ≤ .0052) in use of ADA-compliant grab bars that were available for use with each fixture. Most notably, the prototype with vertical handles which was designed for people who stand to transfer, was associated with highest incidence of handhold use and the lowest incidences of mobility device and grab bar use.

Despite the significant decreases in use of both wmds and wall-mounted, ADA-compliant grab bars, the total number of uses (grab bars + integral handles + wmds) did not differ significantly across fixtures. This suggests that the integral handles were better positioned than either grab bars or wmds to assist at certain stages of the transfer (e.g., lowering down onto the toilet). Moreover, some handholds (particularly, the vertical handles) were better positioned than others.

CONCLUSIONS

The population of people with mobility impairments is aging. This does not mean simply that people who use wheelchairs are simply getting older. Rather, it means that large numbers of people are beginning to use wheelchairs, as well as other mobility aids, as they age. Moreover, many of these older people who are aging into disability are likely to be *wheelchair-assisted* (semiambulatory) rather than *wheelchair-dependent* (nonambulatory). This is an important distinction because people who are wheelchair-assisted tend to use toilets more like ambulatory than nonambulatory individuals.

One consequence of the changing population of people with disabilities is that the preferred ADA configuration clearly does not work as well as it should for the majority of older adults. This includes not only people who stand to transfer, but also those who transfer directly from wheelchair to toilet. In general, subjects who stand to transfer consistently reported that the preferred ADA configuration was the most difficult to use, whereas nonambulatory survey respondents reported that all of the configurations (including the preferred ADA configuration) were equally difficult. These findings were supported by both laboratory studies in which a number of grab bar configurations and toilet mounted handles that did not comply with accessibility codes were found to be less difficult and used more often to provide assistance than the preferred ADA configuration alone.

Findings related to frequency of use of grab bars, integral handles, and mobility aids help to provide a clearer picture of how older people get on and off a toilet. Findings from the two laboratory studies suggest that older people will use whatever device is closest to them, regardless of whether that device was intended to facilitate transfer (e.g., integral handle) or not (e.g., wheelchair). Therefore, the more appropriate the locations of grab bars or handholds the greater the frequency of their use and the lower the frequency of use of wheelchairs to assist with transfer. Conversely, the more inappropriate the location of grab bars or handholds, the lower the frequency of their use and the greater the frequency of use of wheelchairs to assist with transfer. Most importantly, laboratory observations revealed that designs which represented the most radical departures from the accessibility standards (i.e., the swing-away grab bars and toilet prototype with vertical handles) were associated with higher frequencies of grab bar/handhold use and significantly lower frequencies in mobility aid use.

These patterns of grab bar and handhold use raise some important questions concerning the applicability of the ADA configuration in promoting independent toileting by older people with disabilities. Specifically, the preferred ADAAG configuration does not facilitate standing transfers and therefore is considerably more difficult and less safe for older individuals. This may result in higher levels of dependency in toileting than those predicted by clinical assessments of functional capabilities. To reduce these "excess disabilities,"

ADAAG must promote designs that are more responsive to the functional capabilities of older adults.

Clearly, we need to rethink our approach to accessible design from one geared primarily toward young, nonambulatory individuals to one that also effectively addresses the needs of older, mostly ambulatory and semiambulatory individuals. Moreover, to develop ADAAGE, the provision of several alternative designs might be necessary (e.g., a toilet stall with rear and side grab bars as well as one with two side grab bars), to accommodate people who have myriad comorbidities and secondary conditions in conjunction with their primary diagnoses. This approach is particularly important in the design of facilities that will be used mainly by older adults, such as nursing homes and senior centers.

Finally, it should be reiterated that these studies were concerned only with independent transfer, which is the underlying presumption of the ADAAG. Unfortunately, many older people lack the upper body strength to pull themselves out of a wheelchair or have problems raising and lowering themselves onto a toilet even with the assistance of grab bars. Such individuals may require person-assisted transfers, regardless of the grab bar configuration.

NOTES

1. For purposes of the study, this included people who used no aids or walking aids, as well as those who used wheeled mobility devices, but who got out of the chair and stood to transfer.

2. It should be noted that the swing-away grab bar may have received the highest difficulty ratings because it was novel or the plan drawing may not have been comprehensible to many respondents.

REFERENCES

Bureau of the Census. (1983). *Statistical Abstract of the United States, 1982-83, 103rd Edition*. Economics and Statistics Administration, US Department of Commerce.

Bureau of the Census. (1992). *Statistical Abstract of the United States, 1992, 112th Edition*. Economics and Statistics Administration, US Department of Commerce.

Chirikos, T. N. (1986). Accounting for the historical rise in work disability prevalence. *Milbank Memorial Fund Quarterly Healthy and Society, 64*: 271-301.

Colvez, A., & Blanchet, M. (1981). Disability trends in the United States population

1966-76: Analysis of reported causes. *American Journal of Public Health, 71*: 464-471.

Czaja, S. (1984). *Hand Anthropometrics*. Technical paper prepared for the U.S. Architectural and Transportation Barriers Compliance Board. Washington, D.C.

Faletti, M. V. (1984). Human factors research and functional environments for the aged. In I. Altman, M. P. Lawton, and J. F. Wohlwill (Eds.), *Elderly People and the Environment*. New York: Plenum Press.

Jones, M. L. & Sanford, J. A. (1996). People with mobility impairments in the United States today and in 2010. *Assistive Technology, 7*(2).

Kunkel, S. R. & Applebaum, R. A. (1992). Estimating the prevalence of long-term disability for an aging society. *Journal of Gerontology, 47*(5): S253-60, September.

LaPlante, M. P., Hendershot, G. E., & Moss, A. J. (1992). Assistive technology devices and home accessibility features: Prevalence, Payment, Need, and Trends. *Advance Data, No. 217*. National Center for Health Statistics, Centers for Disease Control, Public Health Service, US Department of Health and Human Services.

Lawton, M. P. (1986). *Environment and Aging (2nd Edition)*. Albany, NY: Center for the Study on Aging.

Sanford, J. A., & Megrew, M. B. (1995). An evaluation of grab bars to meet the needs of elderly people. *Assistive Technology, 7*(1), 36-47.

Steinfeld, E. & Shea, S. (1993). Enabling home environments. Identifying barriers to independence. *Technology and Disability, 2*(4), 69-79.

Zola, I. K. (1993). Disability statistics: What we count and what it tells us. *Journal of Disability Policy Studies, 4*(2), 9-39.

A Key to Aging in Place:
Vision Rehabilitation for Older Adults

Cynthia Stuen, DSW
Roxane Offner, MSSW

SUMMARY. Vision impairment is often overlooked by gerontological health professionals or attributed to normal age-related vision changes. With 26% of persons over the age of 75 reporting a vision impairment, it is time for vision rehabilitation professionals to be recognized and included in the multi-disciplinary service team. As the older adult population increases in numbers and longevity increases, it is expected that serious vision loss will become more prevalent. Recognizing the indicators of normal and pathological vision changes and the appropriate individual and environmental intervention strategies available are presented. A functional vision screening questionnaire is offered. Recognition of the unique and complimentary roles of each particular rehabilitation discipline can lead to more effective collaboration. *[Article copies available for a fee from The Haworth Document Delivery Service: 1-800-342-9678. E-mail address: getinfo@haworthpressinc.com <Website: http://www.haworthpressinc.com>]*

KEYWORDS. Vision rehabilitation, age-related vision loss, vision impairment, visual disability, functional vision, vision disorders, excess disability, functional independence, low vision, partial sight, environmental adaptation

---

Cynthia Stuen is Senior Vice President for Education and Director, Lighthouse National Center for Vision and Aging, and Roxane Offner is ADA Consultant, both at Lighthouse International, 111 East 59th Street, New York, NY 10022 (E-mail: cstuen@lighthouse.org).

[Haworth co-indexing entry note]: "A Key to Aging in Place: Vision Rehabilitation for Older Adults." Stuen, Cynthia, and Roxane Offner. Co-published simultaneously in *Physical & Occupational Therapy in Geriatrics* (The Haworth Press, Inc.) Vol. 16, No. 3/4, 1999, pp. 59-77; and: *Aging in Place: Designing, Adapting, and Enhancing the Home Environment* (ed: Ellen D. Taira, and Jodi L. Carlson) The Haworth Press, Inc., 1999, pp. 59-77. Single or multiple copies of this article are available for a fee from The Haworth Document Delivery Service [1-800-342-9678, 9:00 a.m. - 5:00 p.m. (EST). E-mail address: getinfo@haworth pressinc.com].

INTRODUCTION

Knowing that vision rehabilitation is available and how to access it can be the key to maintaining the independence of our burgeoning older adult population in the least restrictive environment. Older adults, being more prone to a multitude of chronic conditions, present a multidisciplinary challenge to professionals. Vision loss is one of the most common and feared conditions of later life. One in six Americans (13.5 million people), 45 years of age and older, report some problem with their vision according to *The Lighthouse National Survey on Vision Loss: The Experience, Attitudes and Knowledge of Middle-aged and Older Americans (1995)*. This national survey, conducted for the Lighthouse by Louis Harris and Associates, was the first ever on the specific topic of age-related vision loss and found vision loss among this population to be much higher than previously estimated. The data from 1,429 Americans age 45 and over, randomly selected for telephone interviews, reveals very high prevalence rates for the population as it ages:

- Age 45 and over: 17% (one in six) report a vision problem
- Age 65 and over: 20% (one in five) report a vision problem
- Age 75 and over: 26% (one in four) report a vision problem

The questions were asked of people living in the community. Respondents were asked to answer the questions in terms of wearing their best eyeglass or contact lens prescription. Since there was no clinical eye exam, some reported vision problems may simply be due to lack of a current or accurate refraction.

Other Lighthouse research studies of older adults residing in nursing home settings have documented that more than 40% of the residents have impaired vision. Too often, the specialized services of vision rehabilitation professionals are not a part of the full rehabilitation team and excess disability prevails because neither the older adult nor the nursing home staff has learned to maximize independence without full vision (Horowitz, 1988; Horowitz et al., 1994; Stuen & Fangmeier, 1994).

As the proportion of the elderly population increases, serious vision loss is expected to become more prevalent (Tielsch, 1994). A study of admissions to a hospital inpatient rehabilitation unit found that almost 6% of the admissions met the criterion of legal blindness and more than two-thirds of that portion were over the age of 65 (Wainapel, 1989). For the population over age 70, vision loss ranks third among chronic conditions, after arthritis and heart disease, that result in a need for assistance with activities of daily living (LaPlante, 1988).

Maximizing functional independence and keeping older adults in a least restrictive environment will necessarily involve vision rehabilitation specialists as part of the gerontological/geriatric multidisciplinary rehabilitation team. Recognizing what aspects of age-related vision loss are normal versus those that are not, who are the specialists involved, and what are the available low-tech and high-tech interventions will be explained in this article.

NORMAL AGE-RELATED VISION CHANGES

Before exploring the more common age-related vision disorders, it is important to note the normal age-related vision changes that occur (Faye & Stuen, 1995). All health and human service providers should keep these changes in mind when designing environments that older adults frequent as there are often simple, low-tech solutions to accommodate normal age-related vision changes.

Anatomic Changes: The cornea generally remains clear, but it may become slightly thicker and more likely to scatter light. The lens invariably becomes denser, more yellow, and less elastic. These changes account for the loss of accommodation (focusing power). The pupil tends to become smaller, permitting less light to be admitted to the eye; hence, the older individual needs more time to adjust to changing levels of illumination (see Figure 1A).

Visual Acuity: Visual acuity is remarkably well preserved in the older adult population according to the Framingham Heart Study that is based upon prospective evaluation of an entire town (Kannel & Gordon, 1973). Corrected visual acuity of at least 20/25 in the better eye is retained by 92% of the individuals between 65 and 74 and 70% between 75 and 85 years of age. However, visual function is dependent on much more than visual acuity.

Accommodation: Presbyopia, or the loss of accommodation, is the most universal age-related ocular deficiency. Sometime in one's 40s, near vision becomes 'out of focus' and optical correction is required with bifocals, trifocals, or reading glasses.

Color and Night Vision: The blue and green end of the color spectrum is more difficult to distinguish than the red/yellow end. Most older individuals adjust more slowly to changes in illumination and are generally able to see less at night than their youthful counterparts.

Contrast and Glare Sensitivity: Generally, older adults have some loss of contrast sensitivity, meaning that they need sharper contrasts and sharper edges in order to discriminate between objects. These difficulties are made worse by increased sensitivity to glare. The thickened cornea or yellowing lens scatters light and interferes with vision; older adults are more susceptible to visual discomfort under bright light conditions or at night with oncoming headlights.

Visual Quality and Lighting: When lighting is optimal for the older adult, normal vision is quite good. However, many older adults experience difficulty performing visual tasks under adverse lighting or changing illumination levels. For these reasons, environmental conditions and lighting are very critical considerations for older adults with normal age-related vision changes.

AGE-RELATED VISION DISORDERS

Vision impairment should be thought of as a continuum, from total blindness at one extreme to varying degrees of partial sight, or low vision, at the other. The World Health Organization officially abandoned the simple dichotomy of vision-blindness in 1975 in its ninth revision of the *International Classification of Diseases*, recognizing that there is a vast gray area between normal vision and blindness, referred to as low vision (Colenbrander & Fletcher, 1995). The type of vision impairment is important to understand as well as its impact on daily function.

Older adults constitute the most vulnerable group for common eye disorders such as cataract, macular degeneration, glaucoma, and diabetic retinopathy. These disorders result in either overall blur, central or peripheral visual field loss. *Low vision* is said to exist when ordinary corrective lenses, medical treatment and/or surgery are unable to correct a person's sight to the normal range. The goal of low vision care and other vision rehabilitation services is to maximize the person's useable sight, and utilization of other sensory functions in combination with adaptive technologies and devices to perform usual, routine tasks. Diminishment of other senses, particularly hearing, in combination with vision loss, may make it even more difficult for the older adult to function independently.

Cataract, the most common age-related eye condition, is a clouding of the normally clear and transparent lens of the eye that reduces passage of light. Everything looks hazy and there is increased sensitiv-

FIGURE 1A. Diagram of the Eye

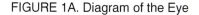

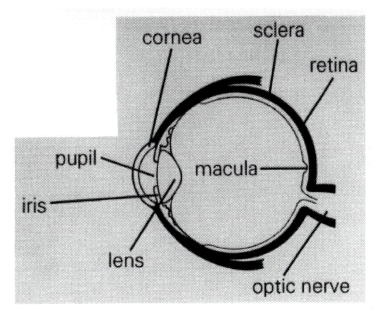

ity to glare. A simulation of blurry vision is seen in Figure 1B. Cataract removal by surgery is recommended when the person's vision has affected the ability to perform everyday tasks. Cataract surgery with a lens implant can restore vision to its former clarity.

Macular degeneration is the leading cause of vision loss among older adults. It is degenerative and causes blurred and distorted central vision; the most common type among older adults is the 'dry' form. Approximately 15 million individuals in the United States have age-related macular degeneration (Chalifoux, 1991). It is estimated that about 16,000 new cases of macular degeneration are diagnosed each year (Egan & Seddon, 1994). Figure 1C simulates the loss of central vision in reading. Scarring occurs in the macular area (the center of the retina) and creates difficulty in reading, writing, sewing, recognizing faces–anything that requires detailed visual work. There is no cure; however, vision rehabilitation can be very effective for learning to cope.

Glaucoma is often referred to as the "sneak thief of sight" because

FIGURE 1B. Blurry Vision, e.g., Cataract

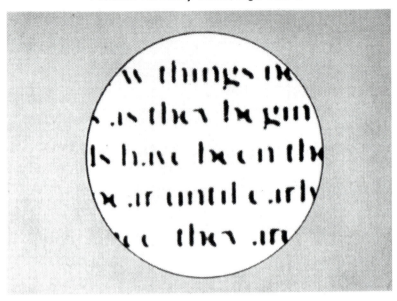

© Lighthouse International

it affects peripheral vision very gradually and can be quite advanced before it is detected. Ordinary open-angle glaucoma affects about 2.5% of the population age 40 and over and increases with age (Marmor, 1995). The condition is treatable and therefore an annual geriatric medical exam should include glaucoma tests performed by an eye care specialist. The loss of peripheral or side vision is simulated in Figure 1D. Early diagnosis and treatment are very important to prevent further loss. Since central vision remains intact, reading is not usually a problem. However, orientation and mobility training is essential.

Diabetic retinopathy results from a complication of diabetes. Good control and management of diabetes can delay the onset, but retinopathy cannot be prevented. There is a breakdown of the blood vessels of the retina. Damaged blood vessels may leak fluid or blood in the eye, which results in retinal scars that distort vision and/or create blind spots (see Figure 1E). A person's vision may fluctuate daily from nearly normal to very blurred, distorted or partially blocked. While vision rehabilitation can contribute to independent visual functioning, controlling diabetes is critical to minimizing its effects on vision.

FIGURE 1C. Central Loss of Vision, e.g., Macular Degeneration

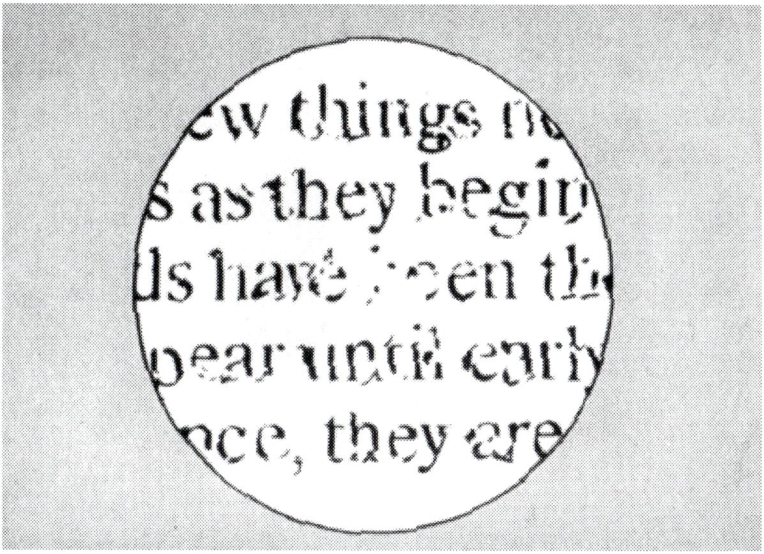

© Lighthouse International

Hemianopia is the loss of half of the visual field in the eye. The degree of visual loss from a major cerebral stroke depends on the area of cortical involvement. The most common defect, homonymous hemianopia, occurs in corresponding halves of the field of vision as shown in Figure 1F. People with hemianopia may find it difficult to find the beginning of a line of print, or bump into objects on one side, and therefore require training to learn to use their reduced field of vision.

HOW TO RECOGNIZE IMPAIRED VISION

There are a number of behavioral cues that can be observed in the older population that may be early signs of impaired vision. The Lighthouse Research Institute developed and validated a fifteen-item Functional Vision Screening Questionnaire (1996) that is very useful to identify functional indicators of vision problems in older adults. The questionnaire, available in seven languages, may be filled out by the older adult or administered by an interviewer and only requires

FIGURE 1D. Peripheral Loss of Vision, e.g., Glaucoma

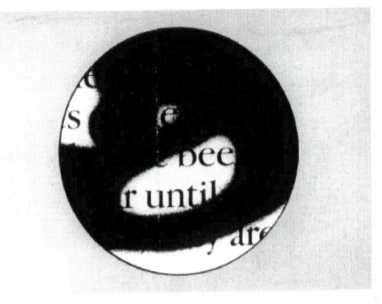

© Lighthouse International

simple yes or no responses. Horowitz (1996) documents that the screening questionnaire is easily understood by older adults and taps areas of daily functioning relevant to vision. Her validation study results indicate that a cut-score of nine (respondents reporting problems in nine of the 15 items) was appropriate for prompt referral for a full eye examination. Some of the behavioral indicators are: unable to find things; unable to read standard newsprint; unable to recognize a friend across the room or the street; and difficulty seeing in dim light or sitting very close to the television. A copy of the questionnaire and instructions for administration are appended.

WHAT IS VISION REHABILITATION?

Vision rehabilitation is a set of restorative services, including low vision assessment and optical aid prescription, training in orientation and mobility, and training in skills of daily living by which people with impaired vision learn or relearn skills. It encompasses a variety of services provided by specially trained professionals to help people

FIGURE 1E. Blind Spots/Distorted Vision, e.g., Diabetic Retinopathy

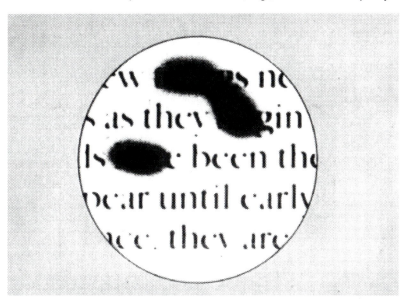

regain their independence, manage their home, take care of personal needs, and participate in work and/or leisure activities.[1]

Low Vision Services consist of assessment and the prescription of optical and adaptive devices by an optometrist or ophthalmologist with specialized training in order to maximize any useable vision. The results of the low vision exam, which includes a full assessment of functional vision loss, contrast sensitivity, field defects, and acuity, will include a determination as to what optical and adaptive devices will be prescribed and instruction in their proper use. For example, some magnifiers require the user to hold the reading material much closer than is customary. If the older person has a tremor, a stand magnifier may be more appropriate. Perhaps a lighted magnifier should be used for certain tasks. Although an older adult with low vision may be prescribed a variety of optical devices, the key to their utilization is to be taught their proper use (D'Allura, 1993; Nilsson, 1990).

Rehabilitation Teaching trains people who are blind or partially sighted to develop adaptive techniques to perform daily living tasks and personal care. For example, a rehabilitation teacher would help the

FIGURE 1F. Major Field Loss, e.g., Hemianopia

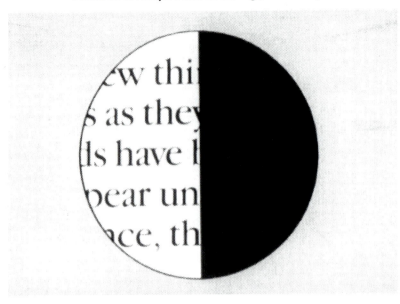

© Lighthouse International

older adult develop a system for labeling clothing and household equipment; for learning to use a stove or tools safely. Persons with impaired vision are taught to use any remaining sight, as well as other senses, and optical and adaptive devices to maintain independence by a specially trained rehabilitation teacher. Large-print cookbooks, playing cards, and address books can make a tremendous difference along with check writing and signature guides, voice-output watches, clocks and thermostats.

Orientation and Mobility Training teaches individuals with vision loss to develop an awareness of themselves in relation to their surroundings and to move and travel safely and independently. People with impaired vision must be taught to gather auditory, tactile, and other sensory data to keep them oriented in space and to master techniques to guard against hazards, e.g., stairs, curbs, vehicles, subways. The techniques are taught by a university-trained orientation and mobility specialist and also encompass traveling with a sighted guide, using a long white cane, or using a guide dog.

Career Services help people retain their jobs or find new employment following vision loss. The services may include counseling, job search strategies, job modifications or training to use adaptive technology and should not be overlooked among older adults. Computer technology has been a boon for helping persons with little or no sight to maintain a job. Adaptations such as computer screen enlargers or voice output computers have made a positive difference for many.

Counseling offers the opportunity to address the emotional impact of vision loss. Be aware that older adults faced with vision loss may experience a range of emotional reactions including grief, anger, fear, depression, confusion and/or loss of control and self-esteem. Especially among older adults, losing one's vision may be one of a series of losses that includes health, spouse, friends, family, and activities.

Studies have shown that people with impaired vision experience a sense of loss, isolation and dependence (Goodman, 1985); feelings of incompetence (Ainlay, 1988); and depression (Horowitz, 1995). It is helpful to explore with the individual how they have coped with other changes in their life. Kleinschmidt (1999) conducted a qualitative study with 12 older adults who had a successful adjustment to vision loss due to macular degeneration. Her subjects identified factors responsible for their adjustment which included a positive outlook on life and a realistic view about limitations that vision loss imposed. Their descriptions supported the various "loss-bereavement-acceptance" models of adjustment to vision loss (Tuttle, 1984).

Involvement of the family in the rehabilitation process is an important component to maximizing vision rehabilitation outcomes, as documented by a three-year research and demonstration project (Stuen, 1999). Support groups, either member or professionally led, have also been found by many to be very helpful because they afford the chance to share coping strategies and mutual support (Stuen, 1991).

ENVIRONMENTAL ADAPTATIONS

Given the normal age-related vision changes and the common age-related vision disorders, there are a variety of good environmental design guidelines that can be helpful to all persons as they age in place. The goal is to make the environment user-friendly and safe. Eye conditions do vary and what may be helpful to one older person may not be to the next, hence in the individual's home environment, ask and experiment with the best adaptive solutions. General guidelines to consider:

- Control lighting in rooms; use shades or blinds to prevent outside light from creating glare.
- "Warm" incandescent lighting is often more comfortable than "cold" fluorescent lighting. Aging eyes need more light; versatility to enhance overall and task lighting is very important.
- Older individuals may become especially sensitive to glare; indoors and outdoors, people may find the use of yellow or amber lenses a big help. A hat with a brim or a visor can be useful.
- For older adults, colors tend to fade. Select colors with good contrast in intensity or lightness, black against white is optimal, especially for signage. Also, paint doorways in a strong contrasting color or select a doorknob in a contrasting color.
- Print involves not only the contrast of the text on the surface but also color, point size (preferably 16 to 18 point), font style (avoid decorative fonts), and letter spacing.
- Bold line paper and a bold, felt tip marker should be used to communicate print messages and reminders, e.g., medications.
- Introduce color contrast in key areas such as kitchen, bathroom, work areas. A contrasting color surface on which to work may make the difference between functional ability and disability.
- Large dial telephones, thermostats, thermometers tend to maximize residual sight.
- Use switches that have distinct positions for "on" and "off." Rocker switches and rheostatic switches are annoying (and a potential safety hazard) because it is impossible to tell whether the device is on or off from the position of the switch. This is particularly important for persons who are blind.
- Install contrasting nosing on the leading edge of the stair.
- Avoid using protruding handles on cabinetry.
- Install strip lighting under counters.
- In the bath, use faucets with separate controls for the hot and cold water, as it is difficult to know whether the water will be hot or cold with the single ball type faucet.
- Install at least one mirror mounted so that it is possible to get very close to it, in order to see to put on makeup and do other grooming tasks.
- Use bright lighting at exterior doors, with motion or sound activated lighting preferred.
- Use lighted keyholes and doorbells.
- Use door thresholds that are flush with the floor to reduce the trip hazard of a conventional raised threshold.

Older adults may experience unnecessary or excess disability if they are unaware that help is available, which is why it is so important for anyone in the field of geriatric rehabilitation to be aware and educated about age-related vision problems. Risk of falling is heightened by a decline in vision function. This would be especially true in poorly illuminated areas. An older adult need not become dependent in the routine tasks of daily living simply due to impaired vision. Vision rehabilitation enables people to learn to do all their necessary work, leisure and daily living tasks in a modified way.

The Lighthouse National Survey on Vision Loss (1995) showed that knowledge about the availability of local vision rehabilitation services is seriously lacking. More than one-third (35%) of middle-aged and older Americans do not know if there are local public or private agencies in their community that provide services for people with vision impairments. This lack of awareness is more pronounced among the older adult population where more than 40% of the sample reported being unaware of vision rehabilitation services.

There is a tendency among the professional community to accept vision impairment as a "normal" part of the aging process and to assume that "nothing more can be done" when vision fails. Vision problems tend to be overlooked and undertreated as a result of this assumption. Many older adults needlessly experience functional disability and a decreased quality of life due to diminished vision.

WHERE TO FIND VISION REHABILITATION SERVICES

Every state has a state office, division or commission that is dedicated to serving the interests of persons with impaired vision. Some provide services directly to people with impaired vision while others contract with private agencies to provide services. In addition to the state offices, there are over 200 private not-for-profit agencies throughout the United States that traditionally have provided vision rehabilitation services. They utilize the vast array of specialists trained in orientation and mobility, rehabilitation teaching, low vision, and counseling and are funded by federal and state sources along with individual charitable giving. This service system is in direct contrast to that of physical and occupational therapies that are typically offered in a medical health care milieu and under the supervision of a physician with reimbursement coming from Medicare, Medicaid and other third party sources.

In 1990, The Health Care Finance Administration approved low vision as a physical impairment appropriate for rehabilitation. This enabled Medicare coverage of rehabilitation services delivered through recognized health care providers including occupational and physical therapists under physician referral and direction. This, however, does not take into account the specialized body of knowledge of vision rehabilitation specialists other than the ophthalmologist or optometrist, who are recognized providers under Medicare.

Intervention in the areas of low vision and blindness requires specialized techniques that are an outgrowth of a specific body of knowledge and skills. This is not to say that an occupational therapist or a physical therapist cannot acquire specialized training in vision rehabilitation. As Lampert and Lapolice (1995) state, occupational therapy models for evaluation of and intervention with the population of older adults with impaired vision have not yet been developed and tested; they go on to recommend collaborative efforts with other disciplines and professionals to insure a comprehensive approach. "Referral to other disciplines such as orientation and mobility specialists and rehabilitation teachers may be an appropriate method of ensuring intervention effectiveness and meeting patient needs" (Lampert & Lapolice, 1995, p. 889).

Given the relatively small number of trained vision rehabilitation specialists, Rogers (1996) advocates for a 'specialist-as-consultant' model based on a successful demonstration project in Kentucky. Forming partnerships with the Area Agencies on Aging and having the vision rehabilitation specialists serve as consultants/trainers to the case managers resulted in improved confidence in performance of ADLs among the older adults with impaired vision.

The 1988 Technology-related Assistance for Individuals with Disabilities Act targeted the needs of people with disabling conditions. An adaptive technology device means any item, piece of equipment or product system that is used to increase, maintain, or improve the functional concerns of persons with disabilities. Each state has a "tech act" program. Older adults are part of the population to be served and are actually considered underserved by the Act (Newroe & Newroe, 1994).

CONCLUSION

Offering/providing vision rehabilitation services enables older adults to avoid excess dependency on family and friends and to learn new ways of doing their daily activities. If intervention is not offered, the older adult may deny the vision problem, withdraw from activities and begin a descending spiral into social isolation.

In addition to adaptive skill acquisition and counseling to help the older person with impaired vision regain their confidence and self-esteem, they often find it very helpful to talk about their vision loss with their peers in support groups. Involvement of the older adult's family is also important so that, as the older adult learns to be more independent, the family supports the independence and overcomes their tendency to be overprotective.

Recognition of the unique and complimentary roles of each particular rehabilitation discipline can lead the way to effective collaboration. The baby boomers are going to start retiring early in the next century. Now is the time to gear the practice of geriatric rehabilitation to include vision rehabilitation as part of the team to meet the growing demand.

NOTE

1. For information on university preparation programs in vision rehabilitation, call Lighthouse International at 1-800-829-0500.

REFERENCES

Ainlay, S. C. (1988). Aging and new vision loss: Disruptions of the here and now. *Journal of Social Issues, 44*, 79-94.

Chalifoux, M. (1991). Macular degeneration: An overview. *Journal of Visual Impairment & Blindness, 85*, 249-252.

D'Allura, T., McInerney, R., & Horowitz, A. (1993). *Lighthouse Low Vision Services: Are They Effective? A Six-Month Follow-Up Evaluation Study.* New York: The Lighthouse Research Institute.

Egan, K. M. & Seddon, J. M. (1994). Age-related macular degeneration: Epidemiology. In D. M. Albert & F. A. Jakobiec (Eds.), *Principles and Practice of Ophthalmology* (pp. 1266-1274). Philadelphia: W. B. Saunders.

Faye, E. E. & Stuen, C. (1995). *The Aging Eye and Low Vision: A Study Guide for Physicians.* New York: The Lighthouse Inc.

Goodman, H. (1985). Serving the elderly blind: A generic approach. *Journal of Gerontological Social Work, 8*, 153-168.

Horowitz, A. (1996). Validation of a functional vision screening questionnaire for older people. In *Proceedings of Vision 96: International Conference on Low Vision*. Madrid, Spain; ONCE (Organización National de Ciegos Españoles).

Horowitz, A. (1995). Aging, vision loss, and depression: A review of the research. *Aging and Vision News* (Lighthouse National Center for Vision and Aging), 7, 1-7.

Horowitz, A. (1988). *The Prevalence and Consequences of Vision Impairment among Nursing Home Residents*. New York: The Lighthouse Inc.

Horowitz, A., Balistreri, E., Stuen, C., & Fangmeier, R. (1994). Vision status and rehabilitation needs among nursing home residents. *Journal of Vision Impairment and Blindness, 89*(1), 7-15.

Kannel, W. B. & Gordon, T. (Eds.) (1973). *The Framingham Heart Study: An epidemiologic investigation of cardiovascular disease* (NIH Publ. No 74-478). Washington, DC: US Government Printing Office.

Kleinschmidt, J. J. (1999). Older adults' perspectives on their successful adjustment to vision loss. *Journal of Vision Impairment and Blindness, 93*(2), 69-81.

Lampert, J. & Lapolice, D. J. (1995). Functional considerations in evaluation and treatment of the client with low vision. *American Journal of Occupational Therapy, 49*(9), 885-890.

Long, R. G. (1992). Summary list of desirable home modifications for persons with low vision and blindness. *Housing Accessibility for Individuals with Visual Impairment and Blindness*. North Carolina: Center for Accessible Design.

Marmor, M. M. (1995). Age-related eye diseases and their effects on visual function. In E. E. Faye and C. S. Stuen (Eds.), *The Aging Eye and Low Vision* (pp. 11-21). New York: The Lighthouse Inc.

Newroe, B. N. & Newroe, K. (1994). Assistive Technology. *Mainstream, 18*(6), 30-34.

Nilsson, U. L. (1990). Visual rehabilitation with and without educational training in the use of optical aides and residual vision: A prospective study of patients with advanced age-related macular degeneration. *Clinical Vision Science, 6,* 3-10.

Rogers, P. (1996). Should vision-related rehabilitation services for older persons be provided exclusively by specialists in the blindness field? *Journal of Vision Impairment and Blindness, 90*(2), 102-104.

Stuen, C. (1999). *Family Involvement: Maximizing Rehabilitation Outcomes for Older Adults with a Disability*. New York: Lighthouse International.

Stuen, C. (1991). *Self Help/Mutual Aid Support Groups for Visually Impaired Older People: A Guide and Directory*. New York: The Lighthouse Inc.

Stuen, C. & Fangmeier, R. (1994). *Field Initiated Research to Evaluate Methods for the Identification and Treatment of Visually Impaired Nursing Home Residents*. Final Report: Part I. New York: The Lighthouse Inc.

The Lighthouse Research Institute. (1995). *The Lighthouse National Survey on Vision Loss: The Experience, Attitudes and Knowledge of Middle-Aged and Older Americans*. New York: The Lighthouse Inc.

Tideiksaar, R. (1995). Avoiding Falls. In E. E. Faye and C. S. Stuen (Eds.), *The Aging Eye and Low Vision* (pp. 55-60). New York: The Lighthouse Inc.

APPENDIX

The Functional Vision Screening Questionnaire

Purpose
The Functional Vision Screening Questionnaire is a screening tool to identify functional indicators of vision problems in older adults. The questionnaire is not a clinical or diagnostic assessment and should not be used to replace one. It identifies older people who may be experiencing a vision problem and who would benefit from seeing an optometrist or ophthalmologist.

Administration
The questionnaire may be filled out by the older adult independently or administered by an interviewer. The questionnaire should be read to the subject, if there are concerns about reading ability or literacy.

Be sure to tell the older adult that all questions should be answered in terms of their best vision; that is, how they see when they are wearing their glasses or contact lenses, if they typically use glasses or contact lenses. This does not include the use of any special low vision devices such as magnifiers or telescopes.

There are 15 questions, all of which can be answered by a simple "yes" or "no."

If the subject answers with some qualifier, e.g. "sometimes," "in bad light," this should be noted on the questionnaire and scored as a problem.

Scoring
A score of "1" is given for each item where a vision problem is reported and "0" if it is not. Scores are indicated next to the answer for each item. Simply add up the scores. Total scores range from 0 to 15.

Interpreting the Results
Based on previous analyses, a score of nine (9) is the base score for identifying an older adult with a potential vision problem. People who score 9 or above on the questionnaire should be encouraged to seek vision evaluation from an optometrist or ophthalmologist.

• All inquiries about The Functional Vision Screening Questionnaire should be sent to:

Amy Horowitz, DSW
Senior Vice President for Research
Lighthouse International
111 East 59th Street
New York, New York 10022
Tel: 212-821-9525
Fax: 212-821-9706
Email: ahorowitz@lighthouse.org

APPENDIX (continued)

The Functional Vision Screening Questionnaire

This is a screening tool to identify older people with a vision problem. People who use glasses or contact lenses should answer the questions in terms of how they see when wearing their glasses or contact lenses. This does not include the use of low vision devices or magnifiers. Read the questions aloud if literacy is a concern.

1. Do you ever feel that problems with your vision make it difficult for you to do the things you would like to do?   1. Yes   0. No

2. Can you see the large print headlines in the newspaper?   0. Yes   1. No

3. Can you see the regular print in newspapers, magazines or books?   0. Yes   1. No

4. Can you see the numbers and names in a telephone directory?   0. Yes   1. No

5. When you are walking in the street, can you see the "walk" sign and street name signs?   0. Yes   1. No

6. When crossing the street, do cars seem to appear very suddenly?   1. Yes   0. No

7. Does trouble with your vision make it difficult for you to watch TV, play cards, do sewing, or any similar type of activity?   1. Yes   0. No

8. Does trouble with your vision make it difficult for you to see labels on medicine bottles?   1. Yes   0. No

9. Does trouble with your vision make it difficult for you to read prices when you shop?   1. Yes   0. No

10. Does trouble with your vision make it difficult for you to read your own mail?   1. Yes   0. No

11. Does trouble with your vision make it difficult for you to read your own handwriting?   1. Yes   0. No

12. Can you recognize the faces of family or friends when they are across an average size room?   0. Yes   1. No

13. Do you have any particular difficulty seeing in dim light?   1. Yes   0. No

14. Do you tend to sit very close to the television?   1. Yes   0. No

15. Has a doctor ever told you that nothing more can be done for your vision?   1. Yes   0. No

Scores are indicated next to the answer for each item. A total score of nine (9) or more indicates the need for a vision examination conducted by an optometrist or ophthalmologist.

- For further information or to order, contact:
  Lighthouse International Information Service
  800-829-0500

Note: Questionnaire available in English, Spanish, Italian, German, French, Polish, and Chinese.

The publication of The Functional Vision Screening Questionnaire was funded in part by a grant from The National Institute on Disability and Rehabilitation Research, U.S. Department of Education, 133A30019.

Reprinted with permission.

Using Home Modifications
to Promote Self-Maintenance
and Mutual Care:
The Case of Old-Age Homes in India

Phoebe S. Liebig, PhD

SUMMARY. Old-age homes, while not a recent phenomenon in India, are growing in number, especially in the southern part of the country. A study of nearly 50 such homes had, as one focus, the extent to which these facilities have modified the physical environment to enable residents to age in place. Not all desirable home modifications (HMs) are widely available; for example, only 25% had special seating in bathing areas, 48% used ramps and 21% employed handrails in hallways and bathing areas. In addition, many HMs are inelegant or primitive by U.S. and European standards, but still provide needed environmental support for residents. These HMs are important to enhance self-maintenance and also to enable residents to help each other. Mutual care helps build and maintain a sense of community, in keeping with Indian traditions of village-level concern for common well-being, and substitutes for small numbers of staff. With huge numbers of Indian elders (c. 170 million) in the next century, greater use of HMs in group homes will be vital to ensure a high quality of life. *[Article copies available for a fee from The Haworth Document Delivery Service: 1-800-342-9678. E-mail address: getinfo@ haworthpressinc.com <Website: http://www.haworthpressinc.com>]*

KEYWORDS. Home modifications, group homes, self-maintenance, mutual care, non-Western cultures

Phoebe S. Liebig is Associate Professor of Gerontology, Andrus Gerontology Center, University of Southern California, Los Angeles, CA 90089-0191.

[Haworth co-indexing entry note]: "Using Home Modifications to Promote Self-Maintenance and Mutual Care: The Case of Old-Age Homes in India." Liebig, Phoebe S. Co-published simultaneously in *Physical & Occupational Therapy in Geriatrics* (The Haworth Press, Inc.) Vol. 16, No. 3/4, 1999, pp. 79-99; and: *Aging in Place: Designing, Adapting, and Enhancing the Home Environment* (ed: Ellen D. Taira, and Jodi L. Carlson) The Haworth Press, Inc., 1999, pp. 79-99. Single or multiple copies of this article are available for a fee from The Haworth Document Delivery Service [1-800-342-9678, 9:00 a.m. - 5:00 p.m. (EST). E-mail address: getinfo@haworthpressinc.com].

INTRODUCTION

Aging in Place and the Environment

The ability to age in place and never move is contingent on the livability of the dwelling in which an older person resides, whether in individual homes and apartments or some form of senior group housing. Livability is determined by "person-environment" fit or the level of "environmental press"–the extent to which surroundings either support or challenge older residents (Lawton & Nahemow, 1973). Thus, for older people, a key issue is whether their housing provides prosthetic, accommodating and humane environments (Kleemeier, 1959; Pastalan, 1990; Tilson, 1990).

Increasingly, environmental adaptations in the residence (or *home modifications* [HMs]) are seen as a means of promoting independence, helping people to age in place and perhaps even reducing the need for or enhancing the effectiveness of caregivers (Pynoos, Cohen, Davis & Bernhardt, 1987; Lanspery, Callahan, Miller & Hyde, 1997). These modifications include hand rails, grab bars, ramps, wide doorways, and seating in showers or bathtubs. A 1992 survey (American Association of Retired Persons, 1993) revealed that 53% of older Americans had made some kind of HM: 17% had installed hand rails or grab bars; 5% had replaced door knobs with lever handles; and 4% had substituted ramps for stairs or had widened doorways. While the need for such HMs is important in senior housing (for example, see Lawton, 1975; Struyk, 1988; Struyk, Turner & Ueno, 1988), the extent to which they are implemented in either large facilities or small group homes is not well documented (for example, see Lanspery, 1997; Morgan, Eckert & Lyon, 1995; Pynoos, Liebig, Overton & Calvert, 1997). Most attention has been focused on HMs in individual dwellings and their impact on individuals or couples.

International Approaches

In the UN-designated International Year of Older Persons (1999), much of what we know today about aging policy and programs has been based on the experiences of developed countries, primarily the United States and European nations. For example, international approaches to housing and long-term care have commanded recent attention, but lack Third World examples (Heumann, 1993; Pynoos & Liebig, 1995; Van Vliet & van Weesap, 1990), except for one very brief overview of old-age homes in India (Ara, 1998). Few examples are drawn from Asia, Africa or Latin America, with the exception of a recent focus on Asian nations (Brink, 1998; Liebig, in press). Similarly, research has been conducted on a variety of housing options, such as small group homes, assisted living and shared housing, in the United States and other nations. But few investigations have focused on the option of adapting single or group homes in either Western or non-Western countries (for example, see Golant, 1992; Pynoos & Liebig, 1995; Regnier, 1994).

Aging research, policy and programs in India are still in their infancy. While there is a growing appreciation of the need to address the issues of an aging Indian society, as attested to by the successful drive in 1998-1999 to develop a National Policy on Aging, most researchers do not have easy access to state-of-the-art research by their Western or Indian colleagues. The majority of Indian practitioners and service providers are even less exposed than researchers to new concepts and best practices from abroad. The eighth national Five-Year Plan, recently completed, sought to underwrite more research activity and to encourage voluntary or non-governmental organizations to provide old-age homes and non-institutional services via grants-in-aid (Shankardass, 1995). Some Indian states also have provided grants for the establishment and maintenance of old-age homes and daycare centers (Kumar, 1998).

Until recently, little research has been conducted on housing for elders, largely because Indian families provide the bulk of care for their older members within the traditional structures of the joint family and co-residence (Cohen, 1998; Dandekar, 1996; Kumar, 1996; Muttagi, 1997; Rajan, Mishra & Sarma, 1996). This traditional approach to elder care is undergoing various stresses and strains due to modernization, changes in women's labor force participation, housing costs (especially in urban areas) and emigration of younger Indians (Gokhale, 1992; Muttagi, 1997; Varadharajan, 1989).

In addition, research on senior housing in India has been impeded because of the difficulty in identifying the existence and location of such homes. Indeed, an accurate census of old age homes is not available. One study enumerated about 350 homes (HelpAge India, 1995; Ara, 1998), another has identified approximately 300 facilities (Bali

Arun, 1994 as per Kumar, 1998) and a 1994 Ministry of Welfare report indicated the provision of assistance to nearly 400 group homes (Kumar, 1998).

Increasingly, old-age homes, home help and other services are coming to be seen as necessary for elders who cannot look after themselves or whose families are incapable of meeting their needs, often because of high rates of poverty nationwide (Gokhale, 1992; Kohli, 1993). Less than 1% of India's more than 70 million persons aged 60 and over live in old-age homes. However, such homes are not a new phenomenon; they have existed since the early 18th century (Nair, 1995) when they were created primarily to care for destitutes, that is, elders who are both poor and have no family to care for them. In the last decade, a new type of facility, the for-pay home, has emerged as a way to meet the needs of a growing number of middle-class elders who, unlike most Indians, often have pensions. Their children have migrated elsewhere in India or to other parts of the world, such as the United States and Dubai and thus are able to provide financial support for the parents. With these changes, somewhat greater interest in conducting studies of old-age homes has arisen (see Dandekar, 1996; Kumar, 1998; Muttagi, 1997; Ramamurti, Jamuna & Reddy, 1997). This research, however, has focused primarily on resident characteristics and life satisfaction and, to a lesser degree, on management and quality issues (Ramamurti et al., 1997; Shankardass, 1995). No studies have examined environmental issues (for some focus on neighborhood location aspects, see Shankardass, 1995) or HMs.

THE STUDY

During four months in 1997-98, the author conducted the first nationwide survey of old-age homes in India. Previous studies had focused on homes in single Indian states, such as Maharashtra and Andhra Pradesh (Dandekar, 1996; Muttagi, 1997; Ramamurti et al., 1997). This study focused on 48 homes in six Indian states (four in the south, one in the west and one in the east) and two Union territories (New Delhi in the north and Pondicherry in the south). These states were chosen because they were thought to have substantial numbers of old-age homes. Unlike earlier studies, this one focused on environmental characteristics of the 48 homes (see Photos 1-12).

PHOTO 1. Old Age Welfare Centre (a Typical Entrance with Locked Gate)

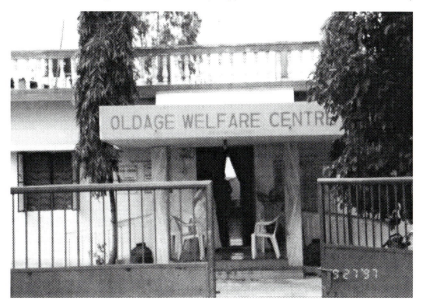

Methods of Procedure

The first task was to identify prospective facilities to be visited. Three directories were used to generate a list of candidate homes (Association for Senior Citizens, 1992; HelpAge India, 1995; Nair, 1995). In each directory, approximately 300-400 homes were listed. The compilation of these directories was based on responses to letters sent to a variety of sources: schools of social work, universities and institutes of social sciences; participants at recent conferences and workshops on aging; heads of senior organizations; and state and national ministries.

Several problems quickly surfaced. First of all, the same home often appeared under one or more names in the three directories; a given home often had more than one address or telephone number. Furthermore, these directories often did not include facilities listed as 1996 and 1997 recipients of grants from the government of India used as the basis for the report by Ramamurti et al. (1997). Thus, a fair amount of time was spent reconciling information from these four sources to generate a list for each state. In narrowing down the numbers of homes

PHOTO 2. Wide Hallways Accommodate Social Exchange and Assistive Devices

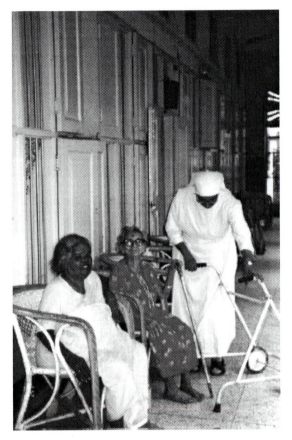

to be visited, care was taken to ensure a mix of facilities according to the following: for-pay, free or both; religious and non-religious auspices; urban and rural (although the majority of homes are in urban areas); gender of residents (male only, female only, or both); and acceptance versus non-acceptance of residents with medical care/constant attendance needs. Homes located in places especially hard to reach were not included.

Second, because the author did not speak any of the 14 major Indian languages, it was necessary to gain local assistance from persons who could speak the regional language. Although English is the *lingua*

PHOTO 3. A Mixed-Resident Home, with a Ramp Going from the Entrance to the Upper Floor

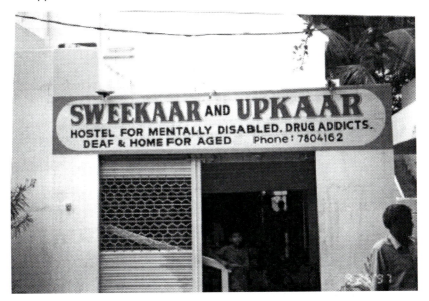

PHOTO 4. A Ramp Entrance to a Cluster of Private Rooms

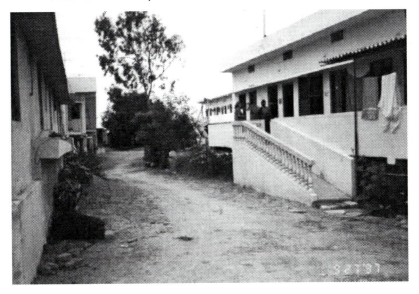

PHOTO 5. A Choice of Ramp or Stairs Provides Access for Destitute Residents

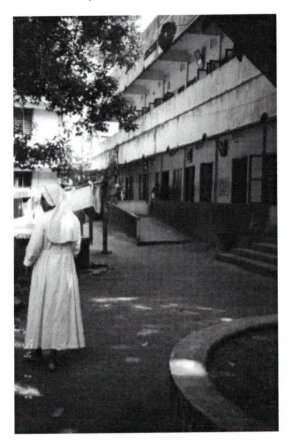

franca for business and professional purposes, help was often required in "translating" the terminology used in the questionnaire and in making it easier for managers with limited English proficiency to respond.

In addition, the facilities that could be visited were often selected on the basis of scheduling, transportation and the ability of the local guide/arranger to make contact with or gain access to a particular facility. Personnel from HelpAge India, an Indian affiliate of the England-based HelpAge International that raises funds and provides grants for programs, were especially helpful. Understandably, the availability of facilities was often contingent on whether the local

PHOTO 6. A Typical Paved Entrance into a Home for the Aged

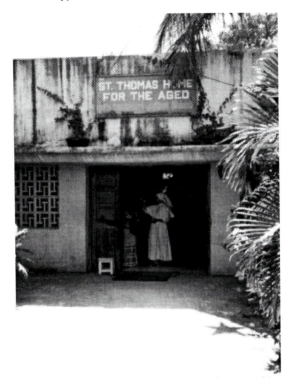

arranger knew a specific facility or was known by its staff. In some cases, facilities refused to participate or permission could not be obtained in a timely fashion. All of these limitations resulted in an opportunitistic sample, rather than a randomized selection of homes to be visited.

Time and travel constraints also dictated how many and what facilities could be visited. India is a large country, ground transportation is very slow by Western standards, and air travel is constrained by the small number of flights available. Demand for existing travel accommodations is extremely high, requiring much advance planning to work out and then adhere to a schedule. Changing plans often in-

PHOTO 7. The Inner Courtyard of a Home for the Aged and the Mentally Impaired

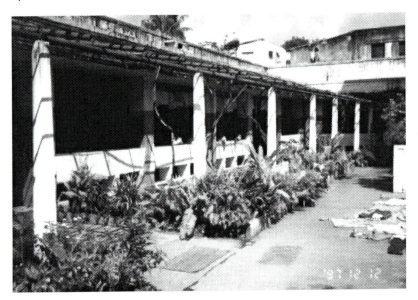

volved several hours of effort just to cancel one set of reservations and confirm another. In particular, visits to rural homes were especially difficult to arrange because of the distances to be covered over poor roads. A trip of four to five hours was often necessary to reach a particular destination, even if made by Jeep. For some visits, budget considerations required the use of three-wheeled, one-cylinder vehicles called auto rickshaws, often rather slow and subject to breakdowns. In several instances, because many sites lacked street numbers or addresses, considerable time was spent in asking for directions and locating the facility.

Each visit consisted of at least two parts: a structured interview of the manager or trustee (and in some cases, several persons participated) based on a questionnaire, and a "walk around" within the facility and its grounds. The latter activity was particularly important in answering the sections of the questionnaire that dealt with environmental issues and most particularly with adaptations that accommodated the frailty of residents. When permitted, numerous photographs were taken of the facilities and often of the residents.

PHOTO 8. Garden Seating Available over Somewhat Rough Terrain

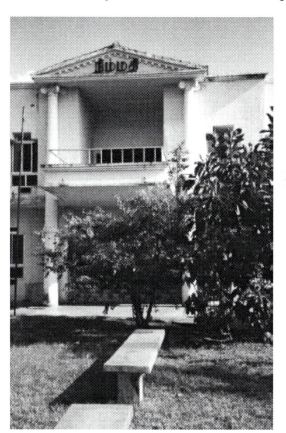

Each visit took a minimum of two hours, but often lasted longer because of the tradition of Indian hospitality that requires the offering (and acceptance) of a meal or tea and snacks. Additionally, residents often wanted to interview the researcher! Sometimes discussions were held in English, but more often involved translation by either the facility manager or trustee, and/or the local arranger.

The questionnaire was based on issues and standards suggested in the Dandekar study of homes in Maharashtra state (1996), the Shankardass·article delineating markers of quality of care (1995), and questions asked by Morgan, Eckert and Lyon (1995) in their study of board and care homes in the United States. The questions dealing with

PHOTO 9. Seating in a Bathing Area (Note the Bucket for Pouring Water over the User)

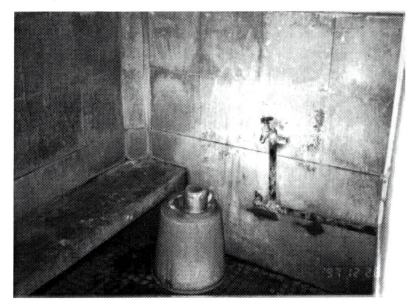

HMs were drawn from Lanspery (1997), Pynoos et al. (1987), and earlier work conducted by the author. Colleagues at the Center for Research on Ageing in Tirupati critiqued the survey instrument and provided advice on vocabulary and syntax that would make sense to those being interviewed. For example, persons who live in old-age homes are called "inmates," not residents, so the wording on the questionnaire was changed accordingly.

Results

General characteristics. Some basic information about these homes is essential to understand the context in which HMs could be found. Half of the homes visited were located in urban areas; 25% were located in rural surroundings, while the other 25% were situated in suburban locations or on the edge of rural areas. One-third were for-pay and 58% were non-pay for destitutes; the remainder were combined for-pay and free. Years of operation ranged from less than four months to 190 years; most facilities had been open from seven to 20 years. Indicating some stability, three-quarters had been operating for

PHOTO 10. A Hybrid Toilet with a Built-In Grab Bar (the "Geezer" Overhead Provides Hot Water on Demand)

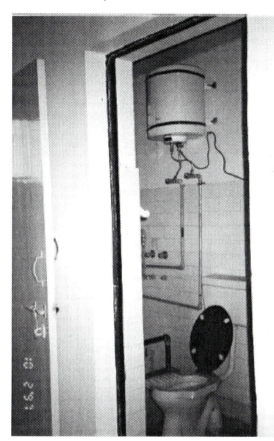

five or more years. In general, homes for the poor tended to be bigger than those occupied by middle- and upper-income residents. The smallest facility had but four occupants; the largest housed 230 persons. Residents ranged in age from 60 years (the normal age for admission) to 105; facilities serving orphans or mentally retarded had younger residents. Regardless of size, most homes were operating at capacity, except for those newly opened. At least 10% of all homes, primarily the largest non-pay facilities, were undergoing expansion or were about to do so.

Sponsorship was split between religious organizations (40%) and

PHOTO 11. A Raised Toilet Seat That Can Be Folded Away

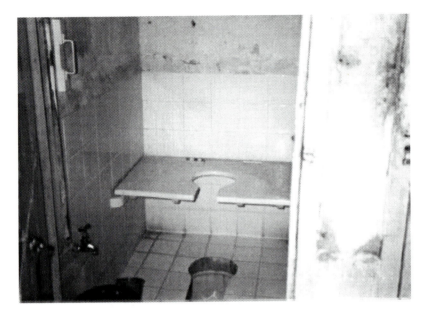

charitable trusts or philanthropic groups, such as Rotary or local women's organizations (60%). With two exceptions, homes were open to all religions and castes. Most homes (83%) were dependent on cash or in-kind donations of foodstuffs, professional services (doctors) or clothing and sometimes even building materials. Their biggest operating expenses were, in order, food; medical supplies, services and medications; staff pay (in several facilities run by religious orders, the nuns are not paid); and building repair and maintenance. Consequently, capital improvements were often targeted on the kitchen (e.g., the installation of solar or steam cookers to cut down on the fuel costs of wood or coal) and the creation of infirmaries. The hand-to-mouth existence of many homes, especially those serving destitutes, precludes their installing features that many managers and trustees sensed would enhance the quality of life and safety of their residents.

Environmental features and modifications. Features common to nearly all homes were locked gates (96%) (see Photo 1) and sliding-lever door fixtures (92%). For safety and security, a substantial majority of these homes (69%) had staff who function as both watchmen and maintenance workers. The door fixtures, standard equipment in many

PHOTO 12. A Grab Bar for Use with a Squat Toilet

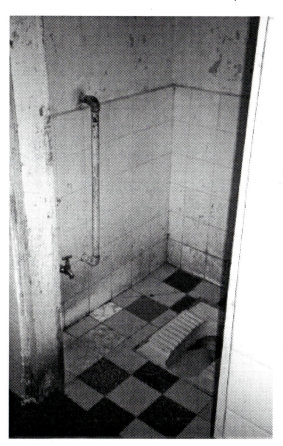

Indian homes, are lightweight and easy to slide, enabling elders with arthritis or other problems of manipulation to gain access to the main entrance or the dining room of the facility. In for-pay homes, this same hardware was installed on the entrances to private or semi-private rooms (doubles or triples) or suites of rooms and could be locked, usually with padlock and key. Non-pay homes customarily have dormitory accommodations, so such fixtures are not needed on internal doors.

Wide hallways were found in most homes (79%) (see Photo 2); wide doors were found less frequently, in slightly more than half of the facilities (54%). However, except in those few homes that were affiliated with a hospital (usually for-pay facilities), few residents used wheelchairs. Indian wheelchairs are smaller scale than those found in the Western world and canes appeared to be the most common ambulation aid; walkers were less customary. The costs of wheelchairs and walkers mean they are out of reach for many facilities, especially those sheltering destitutes, unless such equipment is donated.

Only 21% of the homes had installed handrails in hallways and bathing areas. Interestingly, non-pay homes were more likely to have such features, especially those run by the Little Sisters of the Poor (LSOP). The LSOP homes, which are the closest thing India has to a "chain" of facilities, are known for their high quality and attention to the frailty of their residents. Two LSOP homes and two other homes serving poor elders had installed elevators in their two-story buildings, an enormous undertaking and expense. With one exception, the for-pay homes with more than one story (or 12% of all homes) did not have an elevator; two other for-pay homes had installed a ramp linking the first and second floors (see Photo 3).

Ramps at entrances to the homes were employed by 48% of all facilities (see Photos 4 and 5). Often they were simply hard-packed earth; some were covered with bricks or tiles. Even in facilities with stairs leading into the building, two or three steps were the norm. Many homes, however, did not have level or paved pathways; only 54% had such safety features (see Photo 6). Again, hard-packed earth was customary, whether in the areas leading into the homes or in the open spaces or courtyards found inside many facilities (see Photo 7). Garden areas, found in half of these homes, were often challenging to elders with ambulation problems because they were not level; only 42% of the homes provided places to sit, especially important for residents with diminished strength (see Photo 8).

Rooms for bathing and toileting are separate in Indian old-age homes and are "primitive" by Western standards. Even private bathrooms in middle-class Indian hotels or government guest houses of the kind occupied by the author would be considered pretty bare bones by most Westerners. A majority (80%) of these old-age homes had buckets for bathing purposes, a method requiring bathers to pour water (usually unheated) over themselves, rather than standing under a shower. Only 22% of all the homes provided buckets of hot water; however, in rural and urban low-income Indian homes, cold water bathing is typical. By contrast, for-pay homes had showering facilities, with hot water, largely because the socioeconomic group occupying these homes is likely to be more Westernized.

Regardless of facility type, only 25% of the homes provided seating for frail bathers and no devices were in place to make the lifting of buckets less challenging for older residents with diminished strength (see Photo 9). In addition, shower fixtures were not adapted for persons with arthritis or visual problems. It is not surprising that 73% of these homes reported providing assistance with bathing when the need arises.

The type of toilet found in these homes was not associated with the facility type (free or for-pay). Some homes had only Western style toilets (27%); 29% had Indian-style (squat) toilets; and 38% had both types. One for-pay facility had a hybrid that combined the features of both Western and Indian toilets, including a built-in grab bar; however, its placement made using the toilet as a squat appliance quite problematic (see Photo 10).

Regardless of toilet style, most facilities did not provide grab bars and only one facility had raised toilet seats (see Photos 11 and 12). However, many Indians acknowledge that use of squat toilets without such a support is difficult for frail older persons. Because a water faucet is standard equipment in Indian toileting areas, the water pipe can be used as a grab bar, but not without the possibility of its coming away from the wall. Indian construction is often quite "frail."

It is interesting to note that grab bars are standard equipment in Indian train toilets, to avoid being tossed around while the train is underway. But for the most part, the need for this kind of aid for frail elders has not been understood by managers of old-age homes. At the end of two interviews in for-pay homes, when asked what improvements might be made, the author suggested grab bars in toileting or bathing areas would enable older residents to maintain self-care with dignity and confidence, a goal in keeping with the stated philosophy of 90% of all facilities visited. Personnel of both facilities expressed interest in making these changes.

One startling finding was the extent to which residents are expected not only to maintain themselves commensurate with their physical capacity, but also to provide help to each other; 96% of the facilities reported such expectations. It was not unusual to find residents helping each other in ambulation or transferring activities, bringing food to the more infirm or, in some instances, being "assigned" as a "sitter" or personal care helper to very frail co-residents. In addition, in 69% of these homes residents were expected or urged–their health and energy permitting–to contribute to the welfare of all residents by helping with food preparation, gardening and other domestic tasks; engaging in income-generation activities such as making floral garlands and snacks for sale (23%); and even growing food in kitchen gardens (10%). Only in the purely for-pay homes were such community-sustaining activities not the norm. Environmental features, such as door hardware, level or paved pathways and ramps, enable residents to contribute to the common good and thereby build a sense of community, in keeping with Indian traditions of village-level concern for common well-being.

DISCUSSION

It should be noted that this expectation of mutual care in Indian homes is not seen as exploitation, as it is likely to be in the United States. This is, in part, due to the emphasis in Indian society on the well-being of the group (i.e., the family and community), rather than of the individual (Cohen, 1998). Several managers and trustees also noted the importance of residents being active to avoid depression and to give meaning to life. In a similar fashion, studies of group, foster or communal homes in Europe and the United States (for example, see Golant, 1992; Gottschalk, 1995; Regnier, 1994) corroborate the therapeutic benefits of residents performing everyday activities in noninstitutional environments, adding to their sense of well-being and usefulness.

In old-age homes in India, resident participation in community-sustaining activities also is an economic necessity. Given their hand-to-mouth existence and often the lack or small numbers of paid staff, especially in facilities with religious affiliations, the majority of homes would not be able to provide much assistance to elderly residents without individuals, insofar as they are able, contributing to the welfare of all.

When it comes to creating supportive environments in old-age homes in India, some headway has been made. More, however, needs to be done, as is also true in the United States. No laws in either country require home modifications. The Fair Housing Act and the Americans with Disabilities Act incorporate some rather general accessibility requirements; no Indian legislation even vaguely addresses such an issue, nor is it likely to any time soon. In Europe and the United States, assisted living facilities and their trade organizations (e.g., the Assisted Living Facilities Association of America) are leading the way for industry-driven standards for more supportive environments, especially in purpose-built facilities, but often as a marketing device. The concept of assisted living is just beginning to surface in India; it is not likely to be a dominant approach to housing the elderly for some time to come.

However, senior housing in India is likely to become more important in the future. By the year 2025 it is projected that 167 million Indians will be aged 60 and older, or nearly 10% of all Indians (Rajan & Mishra, 1995). A range of housing options for elders in all economic and family circumstances will need to be developed to meet the needs of this larger older population and their families (Ara, 1998). Similarly, as life expectancy continues to increase in India, the average age of old-age home residents also will rise. To enhance their self-care capacity and ability to help their fellow residents, it will be necessary to pay more attention to their needs for HMs.

The growing numbers of senior advocacy organizations and non-governmental organizations promoting and providing senior housing should be educated about the importance of such modifications in all senior dwellings, whether individual, family or group homes. HelpAge India, in cooperation with the government of India and perhaps state governments, can promote this necessary education and advocacy to ensure a better quality of life for Indian elders in the next millennium.

AUTHOR NOTE

This article is dedicated to Michael Zarky, my colleagues at the Centre for Research on Ageing in Tirupati, and the HelpAge India personnel for their logistical and moral support. Special mention goes to Mr. Vinaya Mehrotra of the Association for Senior Citizens in Mumbai (Bombay). Without his gift in 1994 of the Association's handbook of information about programs for the elderly in India, this study never would have taken place. Research support from the U.S. Fulbright Committee and the Archstone Foundation of California is gratefully acknowledged.

REFERENCES

Ara, S. (1998). Housing facilities for the elderly in India. In S. Brink (Ed.), *Housing older people: An international perspective* (pp. 87-93). New Brunswick, NJ: Transaction Publishers.

American Association of Retired Persons. (1992). *Understanding senior housing for the 1990's*. Washington, DC: Author.

Association for Senior Citizens. (1992). *Senior citizens in India: A handbook of information*. Bombay: Author.

Brink, S. (1998). Overview: The greying of our communities worldwide. In S. Brink (Ed.) *Housing older people: An international perspective* (pp. 1-20). New Brunswick, NJ: Transaction Publishers.

Cohen, L. (1998). *No aging in India: Alzheimer's, the bad family, and other modern things*. Berkeley: University of California Press.

Dandekar, K. (1996). *The elderly in India*. New Delhi: Sage.

Gokhale, S. D. (1992). Toward productive & participatory aging in India. *Caring*, 86-89.

Golant, S. M. (1992). *Housing America's elderly: Many possibilities, few choices*. Newbury Park, CA: Sage.

HelpAge India. (1995). *Directory of oldage homes in India*. New Delhi: Author.

Heumann, L. F. (1992). *Aging in place with dignity: International solutions relating to the low income and frail elderly*. Westport, CT: Praeger.

Kleemeier, R. W. (1959). Behavior and organization of the bodily and external environment. In J. E. Birren (Ed.), *Handbook of aging and the individual: Psychological and biological aspects* (pp. 400-441). Chicago: University of Chicago Press.

Kohli, D. R. (1993, March). Living old age with dignity in India. *Ageing International*, 20-21.

Kumar, V. (Ed.) (1996). *Aging: Indian perspectives and global scenario*. Proceedings of the International Symposium on Gerontology and Seventh of the Association of Gerontology (India). New Delhi: Association of Gerontology (India).

Kumar, S. V. (1998). Responses to the issues of ageing: The Indian scenario. *Bold, 8* (3), 7-26.

Lanspery, S. (1997). Adapting subsidized housing: The experience of the supportive services program in senior housing. In S. Lanspery & J. Hyde (Eds.), *Staying put: Adapting the places instead of the people* (pp. 207-220). Amityville, NY: Baywood.

Lanspery, S., Callahan, J. J., Miller, J. R., & Hyde, J. (1997). Introduction: Staying put. In S. Lanspery & J. Hyde (Eds.), *Staying put: Adapting the places instead of the people* (pp. 1- 22). Amityville, NY: Baywood.

Lawton, M. P. (1975). *Planning and managing housing for the elderly*. New York: John Wiley and Sons.

Lawton, M. P., & Nahemow, L. (1973). Ecology and the aging process. In C. Eisdorfer & M. P. Lawton (Eds.), *The psychology of adult development and aging* (pp. 619-674). Washington, DC: American Psychological Association.

Liebig, P. S. (in press). International perspectives on housing frail elders. *Journal of Architecture and Planning Research*.

Morgan, L. A., Eckert, J. K., & Lyon, S. M. (1995). *Small board-and-care homes: Residential care in transition*. Baltimore: Johns Hopkins University Press.

Muttagi, P. K. (1997). *Aging issues and old age care*. New Delhi: Classical Publishing Company.

Nair, T. K. (1995). *Care of the elderly: Directory of organisations caring for the eldery in India*. Madras: Center for the Welfare of the Aged.

Pastalan, L. A. (1990). Designing a humane environment for the frail elderly. In D. Tilson (Ed.), *Aging in place: Supporting the frail elderly in residential environments* (pp. 273-285). Glenview, IL: Scott, Foresman.

Pynoos, J., Cohen, E., Davis, L. J., & Bernhardt, S. (1987). Home modifications: Improvements that extend independence. In V. Regnier & J. Pynoos (Eds.), *Housing the aged: Design directives and policy considerations* (pp. 277-303). New York: Elsevier.

Pynoos, J., & Liebig, P. S. (Eds.) (1995). *Housing frail elders: International policies, perspectives, and prospects.* Baltimore: Johns Hopkins University Press.

Pynoos, J., Liebig, P. S., Overton, J., & Calvert, E. (1997). The delivery of home modification and repair services. In S. Lanspery & J. Hyde (Eds.), *Staying put: Adapting the places instead of the people* (pp. 171-192). Amityville, NY: Baywood.

Rajan, S. I., & Mishra, U. S. (1995). Defining old age: An Indian assessment. *Bold, 5* (4), 31-35.

Rajan, S. I., Mishra, U. S., & Sarma, P. S. (1996). *A survey of elderly in India.* Trivandrum, India: Centre for Development Studies.

Ramamurti, P. V., Jamuna, D., & Reddy, L. K. (1997). *Evaluation of old-age homes and day care centres in Andhra Pradesh: A report to the government of India.* Tirupati, India: Centre for Research on Ageing.

Regnier, V. A. (1994). *Assisted living housing for the elderly: Design innovations from the United States and Europe.* New York: Van Nostrand Reinhold.

Shankardass, M. K. (1995). Towards the welfare of the elderly in India. *Bold, 5,* 25-30.

Struyk, R. (1988). Current and emerging issues in housing environments for the elderly. In *The social and built environment in an older society* (pp. 134-168). Washington, DC: National Academy Press.

Struyk, R., Turner, M., & Ueno, M. (1988). *Future U.S. housing policy: Meeting the demographic challenge.* Washington, DC: Urban Institute.

Tilson, D. (Ed.) (1990). *Aging in place: Supporting the frail elderly in residential environments.* Glenview, IL: Scott, Foresman.

Van Vliet, W. & van Weesap, J. (Eds.) (1990). *Government and housing: Developments in seven countries.* Newbury Park, CA: Sage.

Varadharajan, D. (1989). Elderly in the changing Indian family. In T. K. Nair & K. V. Ramana (Eds.), *Ageing and welfare of the elderly in India* (pp. 19-30). Madras: Madras Institute on Ageing.

Does Quality of Life
Vary with Different Types of Housing
Among Older Persons?
A Pilot Study

Patricia A. Crist, PhD, OTR/L, FAOTA

SUMMARY. With the increasing number of persons who are elderly, identification of the characteristics of optimal housing that contribute to meeting the various needs of older persons is essential. A pilot study to identify the effects of three different housing environments (personal dwellings, specialized housing and nursing homes) on reported quality of life was conducted, using the *Flanagan Quality of Life Scale* plus two general health items, among persons over the age of 65 (n = 87). Significant differences were found in several quality of life issues related to relationships and satisfaction with life. Persons in specialized housing consistently reported good quality of life related to socialization. While individuals in each group reported no difference in the importance of each quality of life factor, individuals in the nursing home consistently

Patricia A. Crist is Chair and Professor, Department of Occupational Therapy, John G. Rangos, Sr., School of Health Sciences, Duquesne University, 600 Forbes Avenue, Pittsburgh, PA 15282-0001 (E-mail: crist@duq2.cc.duq.edu).

The author wishes to recognize a special group of occupational therapists: Trish Coffin, Anna Lisa Wolfe, and Susan Leeds along with Sandra Marlin and Niti Khurana who contributed to a phase of this project as graduate students.

This project was a learning activity completed by the Class of 1995, the second graduating class from Duquesne University, Pittsburgh, PA, to practice skills learned during their Clinical Research Procedures class taught by the author. Their energy gathered the literature and data reported here.

[Haworth co-indexing entry note]: "Does Quality of Life Vary with Different Types of Housing Among Older Persons? A Pilot Study." Crist, Patricia A. Co-published simultaneously in *Physical & Occupational Therapy in Geriatrics* (The Haworth Press, Inc.) Vol. 16, No. 3/4, 1999, pp. 101-116; and: *Aging in Place: Designing, Adapting, and Enhancing the Home Environment* (ed: Ellen D. Taira, and Jodi L. Carlson) The Haworth Press, Inc., 1999, pp. 101-116. Single or multiple copies of this article are available for a fee from The Haworth Document Delivery Service [1-800-342-9678, 9:00 a.m. - 5:00 p.m. (EST). E-mail address: getinfo@haworthpressinc.com].

101

reported the lowest quality of life. The implication of this study for housing placement, transition, planning, and creating housing contexts that promote quality of life are discussed. *[Article copies available for a fee from The Haworth Document Delivery Service: 1-800-342-9678. E-mail address: getinfo@haworthpressinc.com <Website: http://www.haworthpressinc.com>]*

KEYWORDS. Quality of life, housing, older persons, elderly

INTRODUCTION

'Quality of life' is defined as the degree of gratification perceived from one's contextual experience, including composite satisfaction with physical, emotional, social and spiritual environmental conditions. Quality of life is an important issue among older persons in the United States. By 2000, older persons will grow to 13% of the population and continue to increase to 20% of the population by the year 2030 (U.S. Bureau of the Census and the National Center for Health Statistics, 1998). Not only is the number of older persons over the age of 65 increasing, the older population is itself growing older. In 1997, the 65-74 age group was eight times larger than in 1900 (18.5 million), but the 75-84 group was 16 times larger (11.7 million) and the 85+ group was 31 times larger (3.9 million) (U.S. Bureau of the Census and the National Center for Health Statistics, 1998). Successful adaptation to aging includes preserving independence, which is a major contributor to well being and optimal quality of life.

While the total number of older individuals in long-term nursing homes increases, a survey of persons over the age of 60 reflects the national attitude that most older individuals prefer to have paid caregivers or relatives assist them to remain in their own homes (McAuley & Bleiszner, 1985). Research in gerontology includes the identification of variables that relate to, affect or even predict the quality of life for the elderly with a frequently mentioned one being 'choice of housing' (Clark, 1991; Thomas, 1988).

Identification of the characteristics of optimal housing that contribute to quality of life of older persons is essential. By identifying the reported quality of life perceived through various housing options for seniors, occupational and physical therapists can assist these individuals to successfully adapt to their changing life situations and abilities.

The purpose of this pilot study was to identify the effects of three housing environments on reported quality of life among persons over the age of 65. The three types of typical housing contexts for the elderly were personal dwelling, specialized housing, and nursing home. This project investigated the quality of life factors reported by persons living in each of these typical housing contexts. Occupational therapy and physical therapy practitioners, as well as other health care providers may be able to use this information to 'match' housing resources with individuals in order to support functional adaptation to aging and promote quality of life.

Quality of Life Literature Review

A variety of definitions and measurements regarding quality of life exist, and the struggle with the definition and measurement of this construct continues (Moore, Newsome, Payne & Tiansawad, 1993). Quality of life is defined as the sense of satisfaction and well being that an individual feels about life, encompassing the degree to which one successfully accomplishes one's desires (Gersen, 1976). Another definition reflects the degree that a person's hopes are matched and fulfilled by a particular experience (Calman, 1984). The description of the quality of life experience includes both objective conditions and subjective evaluation of these conditions (George and Bearson, 1980). For older persons, the quality of life construct suggests there is more to life than simply survival (Clark, 1991).

Studies of quality of life have generated information regarding quality of life as one ages. Flanagan (1978) studied 6,500 critical incident reports from adults to identify the major factors affecting quality of life among adult Americans representing a wide range of socioeconomic levels. The results identified incidents and activities that made a difference in quality of life. In 1978, Flanagan reported a national survey of 1000 cohorts representing ages 30, 50 and 70 and found three factors relevant to quality of life: (a) material comforts, work and health; (b) intimacy including friends and socialization op-portunities; and (c) opportunities to use cognitive capabilities and creative expression.

In 1982, Flanagan completed an extensive survey of quality of life among the elderly. Four major categories were identified to describe the quality of life variables related to aging processes: (a) physical and material wellbeing; (b) relations with other people; (c) personal devel-opment and fulfillment; and (d) recreation. Flanagan's work with the elderly focused on differences between age groups and socioeconomic levels but not on quality of life as a function of current living environments.

Social Support Contributing to Quality of Life

Housing provides access to different levels of social support and contact. Clark (1991) states that the importance of social support is a prevailing theme discussed in gerontological research. Moos (1980) indicates that satisfaction with social support and the encouragement to be self-sufficient and independent are related to well being in this population more so than the number of social ties or frequency of social interaction. Burbank (1992) found that 57% of the older persons in their study reported that relationships were most important followed by religion (13%) and service (12%). Less frequently cited categories included satisfaction in living and personal growth, health, income and learning. Since housing creates access to various social conditions, it may also influence quality of life among the elderly.

Housing

Theoretical conceptions of person-environment congruence state that behavior and degree of experienced stress are a function of the congruence between how well personal needs are met by environmental resources and the degree of personal competence supported within a given environment (Lewin, 1951; Kahana, 1974; Harel, 1981; Lawton, 1982). Moos and Lemke (1986) feel that specialized residential settings influence individual motivation to adapt and cope as well as influence outcomes such as a person's health, morale, well being and level of functioning. Since multiple life changes are encountered as one grows older, understanding the impact of housing environments is essential (Clark, 1991; Thomas, 1988).

Various types of residential facilities for older persons have distinct characteristics which result in specific contextual resources (Elwell, 1984). In a recent longitudinal study of living arrangements among older, non-married parents, Spitze, Logan and Robinson (1992) investigated the transitions of living alone, living with children, living with others and institutionalization. Predictors of increased quality of life included opportunities for co-residence, availability of resources, and responsiveness to personal needs and individual attitudes.

Certainly, the quality of life resulting from housing types reflects a combination of: (1) personal choice of current housing; (2) the match between personal autonomy or independence with housing resources; and (3) social support provided to maintain residence in a specific housing type. Living in one's home or personal dwelling should provide the highest degree of personal autonomy and access to resources of all types. Research indicates that independent living promotes life satisfaction, health, and self-esteem (Thomas, 1988; Smits & Kee, 1992; Gould, 1992). Specialized housing such as senior housing complexes have minimal professional staff support, but allow the elderly to retain autonomy and independent living. In addition, specialized housing provides increased access to social activity due to proximity of resources with similar age-mates. Long-term nursing care facilities such as nursing homes are purported to limit personal autonomy the most, not only due to the needs of the residents but also due to a perceived loss of independence (Clark & Bowling, 1990) and lowered expectations of control over their environment (Abel & Hayslip, 1987). On the one hand, long-term care facilities provide structured, monitored social support to maintain temporal adaptation, health, and wellness. However, studies of institutionalized elderly also reveal that residents have limited control over daily activities and lack opportunities for decision-making and creative expression (Cox, Kaeser, Montgomery & Marion, 1991).

The impact of different living arrangements on health, morale and productivity is evident. While quality of life variables have been studied within a given housing context, comparative studies across several housing types used by older persons has not been reported. Thus, understanding quality of life resulting from living in different housing contexts is important to practitioners who focus on independence and well being.

The purpose of this pilot study was to differentiate and compare reported quality of life based on current housing situations among the elderly. The hypothesis for this pilot study would be that quality of life positively correlates with increased independence in housing. Personal dwellers would report the highest quality of life and nursing home dwellers the lowest. A competing hypothesis might be that if one's abilities were matched to the most appropriate housing, a higher quality of life might result regardless of the housing type. Consequently, each setting might support a different configuration of quality of life among housing types unless 'person-environment match' is occurring and 'washes out' the reported differences. Socialization and autonomous decision-making will be important quality of life variables to study. In addition, information on the reported importance related to quality of life components is relevant to better understand the 'person-housing match.'

METHODOLOGY

Quality of life factors, as well as the reported importance of each factor unique to three different living environments (personal dwelling, specialized housing, and nursing home) among older individuals were studied. The results describe quality of life among individuals residing in each of these housing types and initiate a description of which quality of life attributes were most important to the group as a whole.

Subjects: A convenience sample of eighty-seven subjects completed the study. To participate in this study, the subject had to be at least 65 years old and must have resided in the current housing for six months or longer. Criterion on length of housing was utilized to ensure sufficient familiarity with the setting to report one's quality of life. An assumption was made that if an individual resides in a specific place for an extended period of time, abilities and needs must be congruent with environmental resources. In other words, a 'person-housing match' is occurring.

Due to the nature of the study, formal pre-screening for performance problems was not possible. If during data collection, subjects were observed by the researcher as experiencing difficulty completing the survey instrument or responding to initial questions, the survey was discontinued to avoid misinformation. For individuals with low vision, the researchers read the survey items and marked their responses. Demographic characteristics for each group are summarized in Table 1.

Females, retired and living on social security benefits, comprised the majority of subjects for all groups. Most subjects in personal dwellings were married compared to the other two types of housing, which consisted of widows or widowers.

Instruments: The *Flanagan Quality of Life Survey* (Flanagan & Russ-Eft, 1975) is an objective, empirically based set of 15 quality of

TABLE 1. Quality of Life by Housing Type: Demographic Information Summary

Variables	Personal Dwelling Group 1 n = 32 percentage	Specialized Housing Group 2 n = 30 percentage	Nursing Home Group 3 n = 25 percentage
Gender			
Male	22	10	32
Female	78	90	68
Marital Status			
Single	0	7	20
Married	53	10	4
Widowed	44	73	68
Divorced	3	10	8
Retired			
Yes	93	100	100
No	7	0	0
Sources of Income*			
Social Security	63	97	80
Retirement/Pension	34	23	32
Personal Savings	41	3	0
Medicaid	0	0	4
Family Assistance	3	7	8
Two or more sources of income	31	37	28
Living Arrangements			
Alone/no roommate	41	83	56
Roommate	0	0	44
Spouse	53	7	0
Family	6	10	0

* Subjects listed more than one source of income. Therefore, each of these calculations is based on the percentage of the total group who responded to them.

life domains for older persons. Responses are grouped into four categories: physical and material well being, relations with other people, personal development and fulfillment, and recreation. Based on the literature review, two additional categories viewed as important to this study were added, namely: assessment of current housing satisfaction with quality of life and general satisfaction ratings.

Each domain was rated by the subject according to how well the identified need or want was satisfied and secondly, the importance of that domain for each subject's current quality of life. Each domain was rated on a six-point scale, with one being 'need and want extremely well met' or 'extremely important at this time.' A rating of six indicated that the 'need or want was not met at all' or the domain is 'not important at all at this time' for the individual. An Importance Scale, adapting the same arrangement of six-point scale anchors to report importance, was added to the original survey instrument by the author in order to assess 'person-environment match' or congruence for each quality of life domain.

By providing information regarding both satisfaction with current quality of life as well as the relative importance of a specific domain, a description of person-environment congruence could be attained. For instance, highest quality of life could be attributed to items with good person-environment congruence: The domain was well met and rated very important. Low person-environment congruence or low quality of life would be represented by inverse ratings between the two scales when a domain is rated as 'very important' to the individual but the identified 'need or want is not being met well at all.'

Two satisfaction items were added to the survey for this research project to gather information regarding composite or global reported satisfaction 'with today' and 'overall.'

Procedures: As a practical application activity of an introductory research class in occupational therapy, each graduate student contacted three individuals who met the subject selection criteria, one from each housing type: personal dwelling, specialized housing and nursing home. Each subject completed the adapted *Flanagan Quality of Life Survey* followed by an open interview to discuss personal variables contributing to perceived quality of life. The recorded interview data is not reported in this study because uniformity across interviews was not sufficient to draw valid conclusions.

Data collection took place in a convenient location for the individual such as their living quarters, recreation site or shopping mall. The group sizes were not even, as a few students were not able to identify individuals representing a specific housing type.

RESULTS

The median, standard deviation and chi-square results for each quality of life item are reported for "how well needs are met" (Table 2) and how important the quality of life area is to the elderly in the specific housing type (Table 3).

TABLE 2. Quality of Life by Housing Type: Meeting Own Needs and Wants

Item	Personal Dwelling Group 1		Specialized Housing Group 2		Nursing Home Group 3		Chi-Square	Significance
	Median	Variance	Median	Variance	Median	Variance		
Physical and Material Well-Being								
1. Material comforts and financial security	2.053	1.502	2.000	1.362	2.571	1.583	1.9951	0.3688
2. Health and personal safety	1.840	1.246	1.762	1.980	2.077	1.627	0.6439	0.7247
Relationships w/ Others								
3. Participation in public affairs	3.214	2.502	3.500	3.667	4.222	3.277	1.8901	0.3887
4. Helping and encouraging others	2.211	1.064	2.063	1.025	2.545	2.777	2.6867	0.2601
5. Relationship with spouse	1.410	5.444	3.000	5.677	5.684	9.696	11.0071	0.0041*
6. Relationship with close friends	1.799	1.313	1.696	0.741	3.333	2.667	16.2444	0.0003*
7. Family relationships	1.290	0.489	1.240	1.401	2.000	3.090	12.0602	0.0024*
8. Having/rearing children	1.842	3.658	1.500	4.840	4.800	3.723	11.9872	0.0025*
Personal Development and Fulfillment								
9. Learning opportunities and school	3.100	2.667	3.455	3.101	4.444	2.216	4.7017	0.0953
10. Enjoyable and worthwhile work	2.458	1.256	2.182	2.332	4.333	3.623	11.4476	0.0033*
11. Opportunities for expression	3.000	2.161	0.857	1.648	2.571	3.739	0.8147	0.6654
12. Understanding self	2.056	1.070	1.773	0.882	2.400	2.237	3.4898	0.1747
Recreation								
13. Socializing with others	1.586	1.064	1.522	0.805	2.154	1.740	5.5061	0.0637
14. Leisure activities	2.000	1.466	1.682	1.052	2.429	2.807	5.4378	0.0659
15. Participation in recreation	2.867	2.621	2.667	2.882	3.583	3.833	2.7982	0.2468
Housing Self-Assessment								
16. Living conditions	1.333	0.564	1.360	0.687	2.154	2.093	14.0957	0.0009*
17. Opportunities to provide input	3.176	1.797	3.000	2.424	3.000	2.307	0.2507	0.8822
18. Results of input	3.333	2.371	3.000	2.741	3.091	2.777	1.0039	0.6053
Satisfaction								
19. Satisfied with today	1.571	1.172	1.950	1.813	2.667	2.058	9.3191	0.0095*
20. Satisfied overall	1.714	0.502	1.708	0.862	2.353	1.027	6.9782	0.0305*

*$p \le .05$

Significant differences were found for eight needs and three importance items ($p \le .05$).

Reported Quality of Life Results

In the category of relationships with others, as reported in Table 3, four of six issues resulted in significant differences for needs or wants between the three groups: relationship with spouse ($p = .0041$), relationships with close friends ($p = .0003$), family relationships ($p =$

TABLE 3. Quality of Life by Housing Type: Importance Ratings

Item	Personal Dwelling Group 1		Specialized Housing Group 2		Nursing Home Group 3		Chi-Square	Significance
	Median	Variance	Median	Variance	Median	Variance		
Physical and Material Well-Being								
1. Material comforts and financial security	1.952	1.591	1.737	1.209	2.000	1.607	0.9199	0.6313
2. Health and personal safety	1.429	1.176	1.269	0.448	1.429	1.157	1.3754	0.5027
Relationships w/ Others								
3. Participation in public affairs	3.385	2.383	3.444	3.830	3.500	3.510	0.0038	0.9981
4. Helping and encouraging others	1.900	1.063	1.895	1.648	2.091	3.173	0.8705	0.6471
5. Relationship with spouse	1.882	5.868	3.000	5.948	4.500	5.108	1.2508	0.5350
6. Relationship with close friends	1.464	0.641	1.591	0.975	1.875	2.217	3.3571	0.1866
7. Family relationships	1.233	0.338	1.111	0.201	1.350	2.217	3.0282	0.2200
8. Having/rearing children	1.895	4.416	1.688	5.357	3.667	5.375	2.5597	0.2781
Personal Development and Fulfillment								
9. Learning opportunities and school	3.200	2.809	3.000	3.291	3.571	2.955	0.6312	0.7294
10. Enjoyable and worthwhile work	2.471	1.689	2.071	1.742	4.222	3.500	8.4534	0.0146*
11. Opportunities for expression	2.944	1.849	2.675	2.007	2.375	3.307	1.6823	0.4312
12. Understanding self	2.133	1.564	1.762	1.138	2.214	1.202	1.7455	0.4178
Recreation								
13. Socializing with others	1.480	0.752	1.458	0.887	1.875	2.477	8.8118	0.1487
14. Leisure activities	1.833	1.128	1.609	0.778	1.824	2.357	1.4765	0.4779
15. Participation in recreation	2.643	2.475	2.600	2.884	2.857	4.022	0.6612	0.7185
Housing Self-Assessment								
16. Living conditions	1.444	0.656	1.192	0.421	1.571	0.711	5.3300	0.0696
17. Opportunities to provide input	3.563	2.028	2.500	1.828	2.429	1.750	11.2768	0.0036*
18. Results of input	3.750	2.544	2.444	2.893	1.741	2.143	10.8652	0.0044*

*$p \le .05$

.0024), and having/rearing children (p = .0025). Three of the four were significantly different with individuals in specialized housing reporting social relationships with better quality of life from those in personal dwellings. Only 'relationships with spouse' was best when living in own dwelling. However, this may be a sampling artifact as a disparate number of married couples lived in personal dwellings compared to widows and widowers in the other two.

In the category of personal development and fulfillment, the only issue with significant difference across the groups was enjoyable and worthwhile work (p = .0033). The individuals in specialized housing reported the highest quality of life for this variable as well as three of the four items in this category.

In the category of housing self-assessment, living conditions were also an area where significant differences were noted among the three housing types (p = .0009). Personal dwelling subjects reported that living conditions resulted in the best quality of life among the three groups.

Scanning the actual mean scores from this pilot study indicated some potential trends which warrant mentioning. While these findings are interesting, caution should be taken in interpreting non-significant median data. Overall specialized housing residents reported a better quality of life (lowest median) in 16 of 18 measures on the quality of life areas (Table 3) compared with those in personal dwellings. Except for the 'relationships with others' category, personal dwellers were generally most satisfied with their needs being met related to living conditions. The nursing home group's median was invariably below the other two groups as hypothesized except for three items. The items included 'opportunities for expression' (Personal Development Fulfillment Category), and two items under Housing Self Assessment; 'opportunities to provide input' and the 'results from input.' In all three of these categories, nursing home residents reported better quality of life than individuals living in personal dwellings. In other words, living in a personal dwelling limits most opportunities for self-expression and providing input, along with observing results from this input.

Importance Ratings

The participants also rated the degree to which they felt each quality of life issue was important to them. Three areas with significant difference in terms of importance are reported in Table 3. Individuals living in specialized housing reported the highest importance for 'Personal Development and Fulfillment' (p = .0146); however, nursing home residents indicated the most importance for two items: 'opportunities to provide input' (p = .0036) and 'results of input' (p = .0044). Due to the low percentage of significant differences on the importance scale across 20 variables, caution in interpretation is warranted.

Overall, comparing medians across all variables shows that specialized housing residents reported the greatest importance for 15 of 18 ratings. Personal dwellers reported the other three: 'participation in public affairs' and 'relationships with spouse' as well as close friends– all in the 'Relationships with Others' domain.

Overall Life Satisfaction

As seen in Table 2 (items 19 and 20), participants reported a significant difference for satisfaction with their quality of life 'today' as well as 'overall' quality of life across all three groups (p = .0095 and p = .0305, respectively). Interestingly, 'satisfaction with today' was reported as best by the individuals in personal dwellings but 'overall satisfaction' was reported as greatest for individuals in specialized housing. While the groups living in personal dwellings and in specialized housing reported similar ratings, denoting a higher quality of life, the group living in a nursing home reported the lowest quality of life in both areas of satisfaction.

DISCUSSION

The group living in a nursing home was hypothesized to have the lowest quality of life, with that of the group living in specialized housing being slightly higher, while individuals living in personal dwellings would report the highest quality of life. However, this hypothesis was not consistently supported. In fact, specialized housing may facilitate better quality of life than the other two housing types.

Different patterns of meeting quality of life needs among the housing types are evident. Interestingly, regardless of the type of housing one lives in, the reported importance of a quality of life domain is fairly consistent. This may further validate survey items or consistently demonstrate the importance of each in quality of life issues regardless of housing or individual characteristics.

However, two general questions arise, how can a specific housing context best meet those quality of life needs that are reported as most important? For instance, individuals living in nursing homes rate family relationships as the most important factor affecting their quality of life (median = 1.350); however, this need is better met in the other two types of housing. Second, if the housing type is adapted to meet the most important quality of life issues, can satisfaction be improved?

Practitioners need to be aware of the different resources, activity patterns, and interpersonal needs met in specific housing contexts. Likewise, matching individual desires or abilities with the closest type of housing that supports desired quality of life may encourage independence and function. Individuals who are happy with their current situation and have perceived autonomy and self-efficacy to meet their most important needs will likely be healthy, independent and motivated to retain the positive situation. For instance, better 'person-environment match' is found for two variables for nursing home residents: 'opportunities to provide input' and 'results of input.'

The important contribution made by relationships with others must be noted. Clearly, the literature (Flanagan, 1978; Flanagan, 1982) points to socialization as an integral component of quality of life. For individuals with high socialization interests or for whom functioning could best be maintained utilizing engagement in social activities, housing choice can be a very important quality of life factor. Likewise, living independently in a personal dwelling may limit socialization access.

Overall, therapists must look at the disengagement of residents in nursing homes. Certainly some of the reports might be attributed to stigma attached to nursing home quality of life (living conditions: median = 1.571). Importance ratings reflect where practitioners in these settings should focus to improve quality of life: family relationships (median = 1.35), health, personal safety (median = 1.429) and so on. 'Person-environment match' is critical. For instance, nursing home residents report that 'opportunities for input' and the 'results for this input' are very important to them and are moderately well matched in their housing. Reported quality of life seems to result from a 'match' perspective. On the other hand, one is struck with the few mismatches between a small number of quality of life importance ratings and how well needs and wants are being met. For instance, nursing home residents overall report how important close friends are, but how poorly this need is met. This outcome is an example of a 'person-environment mismatch' which warrants attention by practitioners as it may positively impact reported quality of life if enhanced by practitioners.

Occupational and physical therapists who assist individuals transitioning from one housing type to another must consider matching quality of life resources with the needs and even expectations of the individual. Preparation for a change in housing must be proceeded by discussion of quality of life needs and concerns and resultant changes likely to occur. Good 'person-environment match' will maximize individual quality of life.

Lastly, innovative practitioners need to create new contexts within long term care or nursing homes as the needs of these individuals are not being met and satisfaction is very low. For instance, clearly individuals in the nursing home group report that to have relationships with friends is very important (1.875) but this need is not well met (3.333). Potentially creating activities to unite residents with old friends would enhance quality of life. Possibly creating co-op living situations among friends in their own homes or through designated communities would address this need. Another approach might be to improve transportation for seniors to visit each other.

Specialized housing resources have markedly increased in the past two years. From this study, one can see why these environments have been popular. Therapists can use these findings when helping older persons and their families understand the benefits and drawbacks of selecting one housing option over another.

Demystifying the stigma of residing in a nursing home warrants further study. Some of these negative responses might be attributed to a self-fulfilling prophecy. On the other hand, these findings may substantiate reality regarding reported quality of life in nursing homes. Regardless, consumer education and further study to improve the quality of life in nursing home contexts is mandated.

Occupational and physical therapists could advocate for quality of life as influential in health and well being. The three housing groups do not differ in reported importance. However, contexts could be modified by occupational and physical therapists to decrease the discrepancy between importance and meeting needs.

Limitations of the Study

While this study included three types of housing frequently utilized by the elderly, three other prevalent groups were not included: older persons residing with their children, older persons residing with siblings or other elders, and the increasing numbers living in personal care homes. Matching larger groups better in terms of demographic variables would also limit the amount of variance attributed to sampling error. Structured interviews would be useful to uncover additional and contemporary factors that contribute to quality of life.

Future research in occupational and physical therapy needs to further define the construct of 'quality of life' specific to our professional values and philosophical traditions. Professionally relevant and valid measures of this construct need to be developed that are congruent with our service delivery models and provide a unique professional perspective on the quality of life variable (Robnett & Gliner, 1995). In addition, measuring the degree of match between individual performance abilities and housing, which maximizes perceived quality of life through 'aging in place,' is recommended.

If the *Flanagan Survey* is utilized in future studies, dividing combined categories such as 'health and personal safety,' 'helping and encouraging others' and 'enjoyable and worthwhile work' might give a more discrete measure of quality of life in various housings.

Future studies should look at the performance self-efficacy judgements associated with living successfully in particular in various housing types. Self-efficacy can facilitate or hinder engagement in functional activities.

In closing, this pilot study has identified differences in quality of life related to three different types of housing for individuals who are older: personal dwelling; specialized housing; and nursing home. Certainly, more studies extending this information to other housing settings as well as better understanding the 'person-environment match' will assist physical and occupational therapists in providing effective services.

REFERENCES

Abel, B., & Hayslip, B. (1987). Locus of control and retirement preparation. *Journal of Gerontology, 42*, 165-167.

Burbank, P. (1992). An exploratory study: Assessing the meaning in life among older adult clients. *Journal of Gerontological Nursing*, 19-28.

Calman, K. (1984). The quality of life in cancer patients. *Journal of Medical Ethics, 10*, 124.

Clark, P. (1991). Ethical dimensions of quality of life in aging: Autonomy vs. collectivism in the United States and Canada. *The Gerontologist, 31*, 631-639.

Clark, P., & Bowling, A. (1990). Quality of everyday life in long stay institutions for the elderly: An observational study of long stay hospital and nursing home care. *Social Science Medicine, 30*, 1201-1210.

Cox, C., Kaeser, L., Montgomery, A., & Marion, L. (1991). Quality of life nursing care: An experimental trial in long-term care. *Journal of Gerontological Nursing, 17*, 6-11.

Elwell, F. (1984). The effects of ownership in institutionalized services. *The Gerontologist, 24*, 74-88.

Flanagan, J. C. (1978). A research approach to improving our quality of life. *American Psychologist, 33*, 138-147.

Flanagan, J. C. (1982). Measurement of quality of life: Current state of the art. *Archives of Physical and Medical Rehabilitation, 63*, 56-59.

George, L. K. & Bearson, L. (1980). *Quality of life in older persons: Meaning and measurement.* New York: Human Science Press.

Gersen, E. (1976). On the quality of life. *American Society Review, 41*, 793.

Gould, M. (1992). Nursing home elderly: Social-environmental factors. *Journal of Gerontological Nursing, 18*,13-20.

Harel, Z. (1981). Quality of care, congruence, and well-being among the institutionalized aged. *The Gerontologist, 21*, 523-531.

Huss, M., Buckwalter, K., & Stolley, J. (1988). Nursing inpact on life satisfaction. *Journal of Gerontological Nursing, 14*, 31-36.

Kahana, E. (1974). A congruence model of person-environment interactions. In M. P. Lawton, P. G. Windley, & T. O. Byerts (Eds.), *Aging and the Environment: Theoretical Approaches.* New York: Springer.

Lawton, M. (1982). Competence, environmental press and adaptations of older people. In M. P. Lawton, P. G. Windley, & T. O. Byerts (Eds.). *Aging and the Environment: Theoretical Approaches.* New York: Springer.

Lewin, K. (1951). *Field Theory in Social Science.* New York: Harper Publications.

McAuley, W. J., & Bleiszner, R. (1985). Selection of long-term care arrangements by older community residents. *The Gerontologist, 24*, 193-197.

Moore, B. S., Newsome, J. A., Payne, P. L. & Tiansawad, S. (1993). Nursing research: Quality of life and perceived health in the elderly. *Journal of Gerontological Nursing, 19*, 7-14.

Moos, R. (1980). Specialized living environments for older people: A conceptual framework for evaluation. *Journal of Social Sciences, 36*, 75-96.

Moos, R., & Lemke, S. (1986). Quality of residential settings for elderly adults. *Journal of Gerontology, 41*, 268-276.

Robnett, R. H. & Gliner, J. A. (1995). Qual-OT: A quality of life assessment tool. *The Occupational Therapy Journal of Research, 15*, 198-213.

Smits, M. W. & Kee, C. C. (1992). Correlates of self-care among the independent elderly: Self-concept affects well-being. *Journal of Gerontological Nursing, 18*, 8-13.

Spitze, G., Logan, J., & Robinson, J. (1992). Family structure and changes in living arrangements among elderly nonmarried parents. *Journal of Gerontology, 46*, 5289-5295.

Thomas, B. (1988). Self-esteem and life satisfaction. *Journal of Gerontological Nursing, 14*, 25-36.

Maintaining Independence
Through Home Modifications:
A Focus on the Telephone

Angelene N. Cream, BA
Margaret H. Teaford, PhD

SUMMARY. Many different types of activities can be modified or eliminated in order to maintain older adults independently in their homes, but one activity essential to independence, the use of the telephone by older adults, has not been researched.

The purpose of this study is to investigate whether older adults have made changes to their homes in order to make the telephone more accessible and if so, what changes have they made. Reasons for not making modifications are also examined.

The sample included 34 older adults, age 65 and older living alone in the community as homeowners and renters. A questionnaire was administered in the homes of participants for whom information was recorded about telephone location.

The subjects reported making few modifications to their telephone. Most subjects have three to four telephones. The most common technology related to the telephone used by subjects was an answering machine. The study has implications for physical and occupational therapists working with older homeowners who need to modify their homes in or-

Angelene N. Cream is a licensed social worker and a senior occupational therapy student at The Ohio State University. Margaret H. Teaford is Assistant Professor, School of Allied Medical Professions, The Ohio State University. 583 Perry Street, Columbus, OH 43210.

The authors would like to recognize Dr. Larry Sachs and Dr. Jane Case-Smith for their edits of the manuscript.

[Haworth co-indexing entry note]: "Maintaining Independence Through Home Modifications: A Focus on the Telephone." Cream, Angelene N., and Margaret H. Teaford. Co-published simultaneously in *Physical & Occupational Therapy in Geriatrics* (The Haworth Press, Inc.) Vol. 16, No. 3/4, 1999, pp. 117-134; and: *Aging in Place: Designing, Adapting, and Enhancing the Home Environment* (ed: Ellen D. Taira, and Jodi L. Carlson) The Haworth Press, Inc., 1999, pp. 117-134. Single or multiple copies of this article are available for a fee from The Haworth Document Delivery Service [1-800-342-9678, 9:00 a.m. - 5:00 p.m. (EST). E-mail address: getinfo@haworthpressinc.com].

der to continue to live independently. *[Article copies available for a fee from The Haworth Document Delivery Service: 1-800-342-9678. E-mail address: getinfo@haworthpressinc.com <Website: http://www.haworthpressinc.com>]*

KEYWORDS. Home modifications, telephone, older adult, home environment, aging, environmental modification, seniors, adaptations, functional independence, instrumental activity of daily living

As people age, naturally occurring physical changes affect their ability to interact effectively with their home environment. These physical changes are often coupled with an older home that may be in need of repair and presents challenges such as stairs and hard to reach storage areas. In order to maintain their independence in the community, older adults must interact effectively with their home environments. Lawton's (1982) environmental docility hypothesis describes this person-environment interaction as an interplay of competence and environmental press. To avoid negative effect and maladaptive behavior, people must have some challenge or a "just right" amount of press in their environment. Older adults who are unable to make adjustments to their environment may have insufficient environmental press. Most older adults prefer to remain in their homes as long as possible. If older adults are interested in maintaining their independence in the face of diminishing physical capabilities, they must often make modifications to their environment (Czaja, 1993; Gosselin, Robitaille, Trickey, & Maltais, 1993; Pynoos, 1987).

Home modifications can assist people to remain in their homes (Duncan, 1998) by increasing their ability to complete functional tasks independently. It then follows that the scope of physical and occupational therapy practice must expand to include home modifications, particularly therapists working in home health who can assess the fit between the patient and environment. Although both physical and occupational therapists have a unique ability to contribute to the area of home modifications, additional knowledge is necessary for therapists to learn to add home modifications to their practice repertoire.

Many modifications can be made to maintain older adults' independence, but one essential activity is the use of the telephone, along with shopping, managing money, and doing laundry. The telephone is important in emergencies, arranging for in-home care, and socializing with family and friends.

The purpose of the present study was (1) to describe the use and location of the telephone, (2) to determine if older adults have made changes to their homes in order to make the telephone more accessible and, if so, (3) to identify what telephone modifications they have made. Barriers to the use of the telephone and reasons modifications have not been made are identified. The extent to which attempted modifications are effective are also examined. The implications of the results for professionals are discussed.

NEED FOR HOME MODIFICATIONS

Many older adults can remain in their homes if they implement modifications to improve safety, security, and ease of mobility. Reasons for making home modifications include physical changes in the older adult and the overall condition of the house itself. Home modifications may be necessary due to hearing, vision loss, and reduced mobility (Barner, 1991; Czaja, 1993; Gosselin et al., 1993; Pynoos et al., 1987; Trickey et al., 1993).

Home modifications may also be necessary due to safety issues. Home accidents are the fifth leading cause of death for persons 65 and over (Pynoos, 1987). When older adults have difficulty interacting with their environment, they are more prone to falls and burns. Falls often occur as the result of stairs without railings, poor lighting, and clutter (Czaja, 1993; Pynoos et al., 1987).

The condition of the older adult's home may also require that modifications be made. The American Association of Retired Persons (1995) reported that twenty-eight percent of the 60+ population have lived in their current residence more than 30 years. These older homes often do not have first floor bathrooms or laundry facilities, or telephone jacks in each room, features taken for granted in newer homes. In addition to repairs that may be necessary, homes may also require modifications such as adding a ramp or replacing bathroom fixtures to improve accessibility. Since many older adults live on a fixed income, these repairs may be difficult to undertake. There are public programs to assist older adults in modifying their homes, but many either do not qualify or do not know of the programs.

FAILURE TO MODIFY HOMES

Although physical changes, safety issues, and housing conditions create the need for modifications, behavior also plays a role (Gosselin et al., 1993; Pynoos, 1987). According to Lawton (1982), when an older adult demonstrates adaptive behavior in the face of environmental press, he/she will continue to maintain an adequate level of competence; however, at some point, no further changes in behavior can be made or the behavior changes threaten the safety of the person.

Older adults may drastically modify their behavior rather than make physical changes to their homes. An older adult who has trouble walking up the stairs, for example, may decide to discontinue using the upstairs rooms of his/her home. Wylde (1998) reiterates this point by stating that, "Consumers may be unaware of the problems and dangers created by their home because they have gradually adapted their activities and living patterns to accommodate their limitation in ability" (p. 55). Professionals working with older adults can provide information to clients about environmental modifications that improve functioning and promote safety at home.

Gosselin et al. (1993) offered home modifications free of charge to 255 elderly people; 69% had one or more modifications made. Half of the modifications were made to the bathroom (49%), followed equally by the kitchen (15%) and the bedroom (15%) (Trickey et al., 1993). Even though the identification of necessary modifications, cost, and installation were covered by the program, 31% of the older adults offered home modifications did not accept them. A favorable attitude towards home modifications was a strong predictor of accepting home modifications. Other predictors of home modifications found in the Gosselin et al. study included the ability to budget, good housing conditions, and homemaker services.

Another reason modifications are not made is that people grow accustomed to their living conditions and simply accept them (Wylde, 1998). A study by Filion, Wister and Coblentz (1992) determined that of the 280 people over the age of 75 who were surveyed, 90 percent said that they were satisfied or very satisfied with their home and only 14% made any alterations in their homes.

If their recommendations are to be accepted by patients, physical and occupational therapists need to understand the barriers to making modifications and patient views about adopting modifications. Thus, the role of the therapist is critical in assisting older adults to understand the connection between making home modifications and improved functioning and safety resulting from the modifications.

TELEPHONE MODIFICATIONS

Instrumental Activities of Daily Living (IADL) includes the telephone (Axtell, 1993; Gosselin et al., 1993). It is one of the many aspects of a home that can be modified to allow older adults to interact effectively with their home environment (Gosselin et al., 1993; Pynoos et al., 1987; Reschovsky & Newman, 1990; Trickey et al., 1993). Few studies directly explore telephone usage by older adults, although some related studies include older adults. Bowe (1991) surveyed a group of individuals with hearing impairments to determine their desire for new telephone technology services. Only 16% of the subjects were 65 or older and the results were not given by age group. The four services, however, in which over half of all of the respondents were most interested included enhanced 911 services, home security and fire protection, and transcription of speech to text (voice recognition) (Bowe, 1991). Research examining specific aspects of the home environment can be helpful to improve modifications, develop design guidelines, and home evaluation tools (Czaja, 1993; Pynoos, 1987).

METHODOLOGY

Sample

The population targeted for this study includes people who are 60 years of age or older, living alone in the community, and home owners. Subjects were selected to determine how well that individual could handle using the telephone without assistance from another person. According to a 1992 AARP survey, 35% of all older adults live alone and the majority of women age 70-75 are widowed and live alone (54%). These people rely on the telephone for social contact and emergency assistance. Homeowners were selected because they have control over whether or not modifications will be made, whereas renters may not. Additionally, only 15% of the older adult population are renters (AARP, 1995).

Participants were recruited through senior centers, churches, and senior lunch programs. Researchers attended programs at these facilities and spoke briefly asking for volunteers. Subjects were also asked to provide the names of friends and neighbors who might be interested in taking part in the study. Participants were primarily located in three well-established neighborhoods of a central Ohio metropolitan area.

Instrument

The questions used for this study were based on questions from an AARP survey, a home safety check list, and articles on home modifications (AARP, 1995; Bowe, 1991; Czaja, 1993; Pynoos, 1987). The survey was reviewed by a professional working in the field of gerontology. Revisions were made and the survey was pilot tested with seven subjects. After the pilot testing, three additional questions were added to the final survey. The results from the pilot test are included in the final sample since so few changes were made to the final survey.

Questions were asked about the number of telephones owned or leased, the location of the telephones, which one was used most frequently, and the types of telephone such as rotary versus push button and cordless versus stationary. Questions were also asked about telephone technology; subjects were asked if they had an answering machine and if they have any telephone features such as call waiting, voice mail, and caller I.D. If subjects had this technology, they were asked to discuss why they bought it and who may have given them assistance in the purchase.

Questions were also asked about difficulties the subject had in the past year in answering the telephone or making calls and about modifications made to the telephone or that the subject would like to have made. Subjects were asked if they had purchased a new telephone in the past year, to whom they made calls on a weekly basis and from whom they received calls on a weekly basis. Demographic information included health status, living arrangements, recent hospitalization, use of medications, and number of years in the home (see the appendix).

Data Collection

Interview times were arranged with subjects by telephone. To administer the questionnaire, the student researcher made home visits to interview the subjects. As part of the process, observations regarding lighting, place to write messages, and posting of emergency numbers were made about the most frequently used telephone. With permission, pictures of the telephone and area surrounding the telephone were taken.

RESULTS

The sample (N = 34) included 31 women and 3 men; twenty-two (65%) were widowed, and all were Caucasian. The average age was 77, with a range from 59-90 years (see Table 1).

Most subjects reported that their health was either excellent or good (82%) and that their health had stayed the same in the past year (62%). A majority of the subjects (85%) take medication daily and 35% of respondents had been hospitalized overnight in the past year. A few renters were also included in the study and made up 18% of subjects.

TABLE 1. Characteristics of Sample (N = 34)

Characteristics	N	Percentage
Female	31	91%
Male	3	9%
Widowed (all female)	22	65%
Subjects reporting health as either excellent or good in the past year	28	82%
Subjects reporting that their health had stayed the same in the past year	21	62%
Subjects taking medication daily	29	85%
Subjects who were hospitalized at least overnight in the past year	12	35%
Homeowners	28	82%
Renters	6	18%
Annual income less than $20,000	4	12%
Annual income between $20,000-28,000	11	32%
Annual income over $28,000	8	24%
Annual income–no response	11	32%

The average number of years subjects had lived in their home or apartment was 23. The most common annual income reported was $20,000-28,000 (32%), although incomes ranged from $8,000 to 44,000 (see Table 1).

Most of the subjects had 3 (29%) or 4 (35%) telephones. None of the subjects had fewer than two telephones and 6% had 6 telephones. While most subjects had upgraded their telephones, 33% still have a rotary telephone. Only 6% of subjects did not have any push button telephones. A little over half (56%) of the subjects had cordless telephones. Bedrooms are the most common room with a telephone: 85% of subjects had a telephone in this room, followed by the kitchen (71%). The telephone that is used most frequently is located in the kitchen (50%) whereas the bedroom telephone is used the least (3%).

Subjects were asked several questions about the modifications they had made to their telephone. When asked if anyone had suggested they make modifications, subjects reported that no one had suggested modifications. Few modifications were made by the subjects themselves. Two subjects (6%) reported they had increased the volume of the ringer on their telephone and found that to be helpful. One modification regarding the telephone, putting a telephone jack in a room where there is no jack, was mentioned by three (9%) subjects. Subjects were asked if they have the telephone features of call waiting, voice mail, caller I.D. or other telephone features. Only five subjects purchased telephone features. Four people had voice mail and one person had caller ID. None of the subjects had call waiting. Over half of the subjects (59%) had an answering machine. The most common location for the answering machine was the living room (18%) and the kitchen (15%). Reasons given for owning an answering machine were a family member gave it as a gift (29%) and a means of getting messages (18%). Most subjects indicated they had not had any difficulty answering the telephone in the past year (58%), 21% had some difficulty answering the telephone, and 21% did not respond. The most frequently mentioned difficulty was not being able to hear through the telephone (18%). A major frustration in answering the telephone was telemarketers (41%).

Subjects had even fewer problems making calls than answering calls, with 73% saying they had no difficulty making calls in the past year. Only two stated they had difficulty making calls and 21% did not respond. The most frequently mentioned frustration in making calls was telephone menus (26%). Telephone menus are the automated voice information that is heard initially when dialing a business or organization. Several selections are offered and the caller must press a number or other buttons to receive information.

In addition to the survey, observations of the telephone area were made. The purpose of the observation was to see how subjects set up the telephone area, to evaluate its accessibility and to evaluate if modifications would make the telephone more accessible. Most telephone areas were easily accessible (91%), well lit (88%), and had paper and pencil available (85%). People frequently did not have emergency numbers or addresses posted; only 15% had them posted. Most people said they would dial 911 in an emergency, and saw no need to post emergency numbers. Rather than posting these emergency numbers, several subjects (35%) had a personal address book next to the telephone with family, doctor, and other emergency numbers. Telephone books were usually in close proximity (59%), but some people did not have storage space next to the telephone and stored the telephone books in a nearby closet or another room. Many people mentioned that they kept a set of telephone books upstairs as well as downstairs.

DISCUSSION

The results of this study provide a description of how a group of healthy, older adult homeowners use, modify, and locate their telephones. The findings suggest this group made few modifications to their telephones. Although they owned multiple telephones which were easily accessible and used their telephones without difficulty, few barriers to the use of the telephone existed for this group. They reported some frustrations when answering and making calls.

Modifications

Of the few modifications made to the telephone, the two subjects who increased the volume of the ringer on their telephone considered it to be an effective modification. One subject, who has a hearing aid, made an additional modification to her telephone based on a suggestion from her audiologist. Her hearing aids would squeak when she answered the telephone and to remedy this problem, she attached a piece of adhesive foam to the ear piece of the telephone so that the interference was diminished.

None of the subjects said that modifications had been suggested to them nor did any subjects move their telephone. This may be due to the fact that all subjects had two or more telephones. Many subjects stated that they never really thought about having an answering machine until someone in their family, most often a male family member, bought it as a gift and set it up for the subject. Initially skeptical of the answering machine, once subjects received the technology and had it in place, they expressed how much they valued it. When working with older adults, it may be necessary to go beyond simply recommending the purchase of a piece of equipment. It may require that the professional take the time to install it and teach the older adult to use it so the modification will be implemented.

Other than answering machines, the subjects purchased few telephone features. Most subjects stated that they did not purchase telephone technologies because they did not make enough calls to make the expense worthwhile. The older adults interviewed in this study held negative attitudes about call waiting, calling it "rude." These attitudes are important for physical and occupational therapists to take into consideration when making recommendations to older adult patients.

Barriers to the Use of the Telephone

Most subjects in this study were not limited in their use of the telephone by an inability to make or receive telephone calls. They did, however, experience some frustration in making and answering calls. Subjects mentioned feeling annoyed, that their privacy was violated, and meals were interrupted. One subject voiced her frustration about telemarketers by saying that "these people have tons of information about me, but I don't know who they are."

An issue in making calls was telephone menus. Most subjects said that the menu options were presented too rapidly. Subjects mentioned being unsure of what menu option would meet their need and described the experience as "frustrating." Subjects stated that they were not familiar enough with the telephone keys to be able to quickly select the star and pound keys. These issues are important for older adults who often have vision, hearing, mobility, or cognitive difficulties.

Location of the telephone is another barrier, if it is not placed in an accessible area. Subjects had little difficulty answering the telephone. What was interesting about the placement of the telephone was its relationship to use. Although the bedroom was the room that most frequently had a telephone, subjects stated the purpose of this telephone was for "emergencies only." The kitchen telephone is the one that is used most often, which provides insight into an area of the home that older adults tend to use for a diverse range of activities besides cooking.

Reasons Modifications Have Not Been Made

Subjects made few modifications to the telephone. One reason may be because people change behavior before their environment (Wylde, 1998). Lawton's theory of environmental press suggests that as older adults modify their behavior, they may reach a point where they can no longer change their behavior as a substitute for modifications. When this occurs, they may feel that the environmental press is too great and they are not capable of remaining in their home. As Wylde (1998) points out, even if a person experiences overwhelming environmental press, they may not want to use adaptive products if they make the person appear more disabled. In addition, people do not like to be told they must use a certain product or device to remain independent. Professionals must work with their patients and each other to help change the way modifications are viewed. Rather than presenting a modification as something needed because of a problem with the person, it can be presented as a solution to a problem in the environment (Wylde, 1998).

The good health of the subjects may contribute to the fact that few modifications have been made or need to be made to the telephone or home. The frail elderly who are most likely to need modifications were more difficult to recruit because they were not as active. Since subjects were volunteers, recruited from senior groups, they tended to be in good health.

A third reason subjects may not have made modifications is because they considered the modification unnecessary. Subjects lived in their homes an average of 23 years, and may not recognize the house is aging and that they have made adjustments without realizing it. When working with older adults, professionals must consider their homes as a familiar place and that they may have a deep attachment to it.

RECOMMENDATIONS FOR FUTURE RESEARCH

Future research with a more frail population should be done to find out if there is a difference in the amount of modifications made by healthy older adults and those who are more frail. More information is needed about the types of modifications and changes that need to be made by older adults in order to maintain their independence. Understanding modifications and the reasons they are made will help professionals make more thorough home assessments and implement effective interventions.

LIMITATIONS

The subjects interviewed were homogenous. All were Caucasian and all but three were women. A further limitation of the study was its small sample size coupled with the fact that most subjects lived in the same neighborhood and were homeowners. Some of the information gathered in this study, such as ability to answer and make calls, was based on self-report. This study is, however, a starting point for research about older adults and their use of the telephone.

CONCLUSIONS

The results of this study provide information to help physical and occupational therapists gain a greater understanding of older adults' attitudes and behaviors regarding telephone use and home modification. Increased understanding of how IADL's, such as telephone use, contribute to independence will allow therapists to provide better service to their older adult clients.

REFERENCES

American Association of Retired Persons. (1995). Understanding senior housing for the 1990's: Survey of consumer preferences, consensus, and needs. Washington, DC, PF4522 (593)D 13899.

Axtell, L. A. & Yasuda, Y. L. (1993). Assistive devices and home modifications in geriatric rehabilitation. *Geriatric Rehabilitation, 9,* 803-821.

Barner, P. A. & Davis, B. W. (1991). Factors affecting independent living arrangements of frail elderly adults. *Housing and Society, 18*(2), 63-68.

Bowe, F. G. (1991). National survey on telephone services and products: The views of deaf and hard-of-hearing people. *American Annals of the Deaf, 136*, 278-283.

Ciurlia-Guy, E., Cashman, M., & Lewsen, B. (1993). Identifying hearing loss and hearing handicap among chronic care elderly people. *The Gerontologist, 33*, 644-649.

Czaja, S. (1993). Enhancing the home safety of the elderly: Technical and design interventions. In *Life-span design of residential environments for an aging population* (pp. 71-74). Washington DC: AARP.

Duncan, R. (1998). Blueprint for action: The national home modifications action coalition. *Technology & Disability, 8*, 85-89.

Filion, P., Wister, A., & Coblentz, E. J. (1992). Subjective dimensions of environmental adaptation among the elderly: A challenge to models of housing policy. *Journal of Housing for the Elderly, 10*, 3-27.

Gosselin, C., Robitaille, Y., Trickey, F., & Maltais, D. (1993). Factors predicting the implementation of home modifications among elderly people with loss of independence. *Physical & Occupational Therapy in Geriatrics, 12*, 15-27.

Hsueh-Ling, C. (1994). Hearing in the elderly: Relation of hearing loss, loneliness, and self esteem. *Journal of Gerontological Nursing, 20*(6) 22-28.

Larsen, P. D., Hazen, S. E., & Hoot-Martin, J. L. (1997). Assessment and management of sensory loss in elderly patients. *AORN Journal, 65*, 432-437.

Lawton, M. P. (1982). Competence, environmental press, and the adaptation of older people. In M. P. Lawton, P. G. Windley, and T. O. Byerts (Eds.), *Aging and the environment*. New York: Springer Publishing Co.

Pynoos, J., Cohen, E., Davis, L., & Bernhardt, S. (1987). Home modifications: Improvements that extend independence. In V. Regnier and J. Pynoos (Eds.), *Housing the aged* (pp. 277-303). New York, NY: Elsevier.

Reschovsky, J. D., & Newman, S. J. (1990). Adaptations for independent living by older frail households. *The Gerontologist, 30*, 543-552.

Trickey, F., Maltais, D., Gosselin, C., & Robitaille, Y. (1993). Adapting older persons' homes to promote independence. *Physical & Occupational Therapy in Geriatrics, 12*, 1-14.

U.S. Bureau of the Census. (1989). *Current Housing Report*, Series H-170-87-25, *Annual housing survey of Columbus metropolis*. Washington, DC: Government Printing Office.

Wylde, M. A. (1998). Consumer knowledge of home modifications. *Technology & Disability, 8*, 51-68.

APPENDIX

Questionnaire

Number: _____
Date: _____

* How many telephones do you own or lease? _____
* How many are you presently using? _____

* In which rooms are your telephones located?	
a) Living room	
b) Kitchen	
c) Bedroom	
d) Other	

* What other rooms have a telephone jack, but a phone is not hooked up?	
* Are telephone jacks easily accessible or is it necessary to move a piece of heavy furniture to reach the telephone jack?	

* What types of telephones do you own?	
a) Rotary/dial	
b) Push button	
c) Wall/stationary phone	
d) Cordless	
e) Cellular	
f) Other	
* Which telephone do you use most frequently?	

* In the past year have you bought a new telephone?	YES / NO
IF YES REASON:	
a) Old phone was broken; replace	
b) Needed a different type of phone	
c) Needed additional phone	
d) Other	
IF YES:	
• Did you replace the phone with the same type of phone or a different model? (example, replace rotary with push button)	

IF YES:	
• Did you receive assistance from someone else to obtain the phone?	YES / NO
IF YES, from whom did you receive assistance?	
IF YES, TYPE OF ASSISTANCE:	
a) Purchase	
b) Set up	
c) Financial	
d) Other	

* Do you currently have:	If yes, approx. how long
a) Call waiting	
b) Voice mail	
c) Three way calling	
d) Caller ID	
e) Other	
• Why did you purchase phone features?	
IF NO:	
• Have you considered these features and decided not to purchase them?	
• Why?	

* Do you have an answering machine that you use?	YES / NO
IF YES:	
• In what room is the answering machine located?	
IF YES:	
• Which of the following prompted you to purchase an answering machine? (more than one response is permitted)	
a) Not able to get to the phone	
b) Often out so need a way to get messages	
c) Wanted to be able to screen calls	
d) Relative/friend/health care provider suggested it	
e) Someone else bought it for me	
f) Other	

APPENDIX (continued)

In the past year have you been:	
ANSWERING CALLS	
a) Unable to hear ringing of phone	
b) Unable to reach/get to the phone in time	
c) Unable to pick up the phone	
d) Not able to hear what people are saying	
e) Other (telephone frustrations)	
• On a scale from 1 to 5 (1 = very easy; 5 = very difficult) how much difficulty would you say that you have had in answering calls in the past year?	
MAKING CALLS	
• In the past year have you had difficulty . . .	
a) Looking up phone numbers	
b) Determining whom to call	
c) Dialing	
d) Other difficulties making calls	
• On a scale from 1 to 5 (1 = very easy; 5 = very difficult) how much difficulty would you say that you have had in making calls in the past year?	
• Describe any other difficulties you have had with using the telephone?	

* Has anyone ever suggested that you make modifications to the phone?	YES / NO
• If yes, who suggested the modifications?	
• What modifications did they suggest?	
* In the past year have you made any of the following changes?	YES / NO
a) Move location of phone to more convenient location	
b) Turn-up ringer so it is easier to hear	
c) Built up the handle; other modification to pick up the phone more easily	
d) Other	
• Did these changes help?	

* If you wanted to make changes but did not, was it because you found it was . . .	
a) Not needed	
b) Too expensive	
c) Required technical expertise or equipment which is not available to you	
d) Other	

* Are there other areas of your household that you think need to be modified?

    *   Which areas? _____

    *   Describe modifications: _____

* To whom do you make telephone calls on a weekly basis?	
a) Family	
b) Friends	
c) Doctor	
d) Home health aide/home care services	
e) Pharmacist	
f) To order food	
g) To buy products	
h) To get information about social activities	
i) Radio talk shows	
j) Organizations/clubs of which you are a member	
k) Other	

* From whom do you receive telephone calls on a regular basis?	
a) Family	
b) Friends	
c) Doctor	
d) Home health aide/home care services	
e) Pharmacist	
f) Telemarketer	
g) Charity	
h) Organizations/clubs of which you are a member	
i) Other	

APPENDIX (continued)

* Observation of most frequently used phone area:	
a) Well lit	
b) Paper and pencil	
c) Phone cords secure	
d) Easily accessible	
e) Telephone books close	
f) Accessibility of phone jacks	
g) Place to write messages	
h) Emergency numbers posted	
i) Address posted (for 911 calls, etc.)	
j) Other aspects of phone area	
* DEMOGRAPHIC INFORMATION Would you please answer just a few questions about yourself?	
• In what year were you born?	
• Are you currently married, widowed, divorced, separated, or single (never married)?	
• How would you rate your health? Excellent, good, fair, poor	
• In the past year, would you say that your health has improved, stayed the same, or declined?	
• Have you been hospitalized in the past year? YES / NO	
• Do you take medication daily? YES / NO	
• How many people, including yourself, live here?	
• Who else lives here with you?	
• How many years have you lived in this home?	
• How many years have you owned this home?	
• Would you please look at the card and select the LETTER which is closest to your yearly income? Is it A B C D E F G	
• Do you consider yourself to be African-American, White, Asian, or some other race?	
THANK YOU VERY MUCH FOR YOUR TIME	
Interviewer completes:	
• Gender: male / female	
• Housing Type: Single family, double, apartment, other	
• Condition of housing: Exterior	
Interior	

Home Modifications for the Elderly: Implications for the Occupational Therapist

Donald Auriemma, MSEd, OTR/L, BCN
Sharon Faust, MS, OTR/L
Karla Sibrian, COTA
Juan Jimenez, COTA

SUMMARY. With society placing high positive value on independent living for the elderly, the need for home modification is growing. This paper will describe current information as well as psychosocial implications the occupational therapist should consider when collaborating with their elderly clients who wish to remain at home and "age in place." *[Article copies available for a fee from The Haworth Document Delivery Service: 1-800-342-9678. E-mail address: getinfo@haworthpressinc.com <Website: http://www.haworthpressinc.com>]*

KEYWORDS. Architectural barriers, home modifications, assistive devices, independence, aging in place, impairment, elderly, older adults, environmental adaptions, universal design

INTRODUCTION

Society is faced with an elderly population that is increasing. Less than 100 years ago, only one in 25 Americans was over the age of 65.

Donald Auriemma is Assistant Professor, York College, City University of New York, Jamaica, NY 11451. Sharon Faust is Assistant Professor, York College, City University of New York, Jamaica, NY 11451, and Consultant, North Shore-Long Island Jewish Health System, New Hyde Park, NY 11042. Karla Sibrian and Juan Jimenez are affiliated with North Shore-Long Island Jewish Health System, New Hyde Park, NY 11042.

[Haworth co-indexing entry note]: "Home Modifications for the Elderly: Implications for the Occupational Therapist." Auriemma, Donald et al. Co-published simultaneously in *Physical & Occupational Therapy in Geriatrics* (The Haworth Press, Inc.) Vol. 16, No. 3/4, 1999, pp. 135-144; and: *Aging in Place: Designing, Adapting, and Enhancing the Home Environment* (ed: Ellen D. Taira, and Jodi L. Carlson) The Haworth Press, Inc., 1999, pp. 135-144. Single or multiple copies of this article are available for a fee from The Haworth Document Delivery Service [1-800-342-9678, 9:00 a.m. - 5:00 p.m. (EST). E-mail address: getinfo@haworthpressinc.com].

135

Presently individuals over 65 constitute almost 13% of the United States population. It is estimated that by the year 2030 this number will increase to 20% (Aitkens & Finan, 1992). The increase has been attributed to the aging of baby boomers, the growth in immigration to the western world and increased life expectancy resulting from improved medical care (Kendig, 1989; Zola, 1993). The associated need for an increase in home modifications (La Plante, 1997) flows from an aged and impaired population.

The concept of home modification and adaption is not new. In the early 1960's discussion of good design and the use of assistive devices was initiated to enable a person with a physical limitation to cope with the environment more effectively (Lindsley, 1964). Individuals with disabilities have been creative about incorporating new technologies, redesigning their homes and eliminating architectural barriers (Health and Welfare Canada, 1984). Despite the device, design or modification, the primary goal is to adapt the environment to meet the diminishing functional capabilities of the older adult and to allow for independence in the home (Gosselin, Robitaille, Trickey & Maltais, 1993). This paper will discuss the current body of research in the area of home modifications for the elderly population. Also explored are psychosocial implications of adaptions.

HOME MODIFICATION-RATIONALE

Common challenges that occur with aging that are considered part of the natural development process include a decline in physical abilities of vision, hearing, strength, endurance, balance and reaction time as well as cognitive abilities of short term memory, abstraction, mental flexibility, information processing speed and sustained attention (American Psychological Association, 1997). Chronic conditions also increase a person's risk of disability (Mann, 1997). An estimated 80% of the elderly have chronic conditions, 45% of whom have some form of activity limitation due to these chronic conditions (Mann, 1997).

AGING IN PLACE

Current research supports the concept of "aging in place." Though the elderly today have greater housing alternatives available to them, the majority choose to remain in their home (Fillon, Wister & Coblentz, 1992). A 1992 survey by American Association of Retired Persons reported that 84% of people over the age of 55 want to stay in their present home. Nineteen percent of this population have lived in their current residence between 21 and 30 years, and 28% have lived there more than 30 years. Seventy-five percent of the respondents lived in single-family detached homes while 12% live in multi-unit buildings. Fifty-three percent of this population of older Americans reported making modifications to their home or behavior to allow them to remain in their homes (Hettinger, 1996). Older people usually make more positive appraisals of their residential situation than the experts. This may indicate diverging assessment criteria between these two groups (Golant, 1986).

More than 10 million older Americans have difficulty with daily tasks at home (Ringwald, 1988). Even higher numbers have been estimated to need help in household activities in the future (American Association of Retired Persons, 1990). To solve these problems of everyday living the public has turned to architects, engineers, interior designers and urban planners. This group traditionally lacks the knowledge of the functional capacities of the elderly who may also have progressive or chronic disorders. Occupational therapists have been suggested as knowledgeable resource persons (Dahl & Lejnieks, 1990).

Estimates are that 7.1 million people of all ages live in homes with special equipment. Fifty-two percent are over the age of 65. Mobility, vision and hearing devices are more likely to be used by the elderly. One percent of the general population in the U.S. have unmet needs for assistive technology. Forty-five percent of this estimated 2.5 million are 65 years or older. This rate of unmet need increases with age. Forty-seven percent of individuals aged 75 or older have unmet assistive technology needs (La Plointe et al., 1997).

ASSESSMENT

Assessment tools have been designed to help determine the specific requirements for an elderly person to remain safely in their home. Many occupational therapy departments have developed their own non-standardized home assessment checklists (Christian & Baum, 1991; Hayes, 1978; Trombley, 1983). Standardized assessment tools have also been developed. They include the Home Hazards Checklist (Tiderksaar, 1986), the Westmead Home Hazard Assessment (Lettts et al., 1998) and the Safety Assessment of Function and the Environment for Rehabiliation (SAFER Tool) (Clemson, Roland & Cumming, 1992). Clemson, Roland and Cumming (1992) created a study to examine the inter-rater reliability of occupational therapists assessing potential home safety hazards. Their findings indicated that therapists can generally be relied upon to rate potential hazards in the home, but that therapists had poor reliability in assessment of the toilet and shower areas (Clemson, Roland & Cumming, 1992).

Computer technology is also being applied in home modification. Software has been developed for use by occupational therapists who work with elderly persons. One example is Enhancements Adopting Senior Environments (EASE). It identifies potential problems in independent living by comparing functional abilities of the person and the requirements of the home. For each problem confirmed by the occupational therapist, the program presents a variety of solutions including products, ideas, recommendations, adaptions, and suggestions for professional assistance and service (Christenson & Krantz, 1993). To date no reliability values have been reported.

The need to consider home modification most commonly occurs following a discharge from a hospital stay, frequently an inpatient rehabilitation stay. Following an (often brief) inpatient stay, clients may expect to move along the continuum of treatment from home health care to out-patient before they have reached their maximal functional potential. Therapists must start planning for home modifications early in a client's treatment to allow for client and family to make plans for temporary or permanent modifications. Planning for sleeping and bathroom facilities are often the primary concerns (Wright, 1997). Realistically, there may not be enough time to make more permanent changes such as widening doorways, installing a lift, or creating an accessible entrance and exit.

Ramps are used to make the transition from outdoors to indoors. Smolarkiewicz suggests we look at the nature of the older adult's disability. Those who face short term difficulties may chose to rent or install a temporary ramp. Those expected to become progressively worse may need a more elaborate and permanent structure in terms of location and design (Smolarkiewicz, 1998).

SENSORY MODIFICATIONS

Hearing reduction and loss are considerations for modification (Seelman, 1990). Common environmental modifications for persons with hearing impairments have been identified by Shamberg and Shamberg (1996). These include use of telephone devices for the deaf, the use of fax machines, nearby paper and writing implements, vibrating or visual alerting signals on alarm clocks, smoke detectors, telephones and door bells, amplification devices to eliminate background noises and increase volume of desired noise, and furniture arranged to allow individuals to face one another when speaking (Shamberg & Shamberg, 1996).

Environmental modifications for persons with visual impairment have also been identified by Shamberg and Shamberg (1996). These include increasing available lighting, halogen lighting for close up work, adjusting lights for different tasks demands and window treatments that allow light filtering. Other suggestions include color contrast to define objects and spaces, tactile indicators, textures to produce tactile areas, elimination of busy and confusing patterns and elimination of clutter (Shamberg & Shamberg, 1996). Stuen and Offner (1999) have detailed modifications for visual impairments extensively elsewhere in this volume.

COGNITIVE MODIFICATIONS

A decline in sensory and perceptual function is often associated with normal age related changes. The line between pathology and normal aging is increasingly unclear (Lawton, 1985). An approach which promotes adaptation of the environment to capitalize on the clients' inherent strengths and situational advantages should be considered (Niestadt, 1990, p. 299). Design and adaption of older adults' environment is pertinent from the perspective of a variety of disciplines (Roctman, 1993).

Forse (1994) has addressed modifying the home environment for clients with dementia. The following are the recommendations made to improve the physical environment for someone in the early stages of this disease: the use of a well lit environment without glare, the elimination of pictures near outside windows, use of subdued lights in the evening to provide cues for sleep, the use of a nightlight at night in essential areas, the use of contrast materials to identify where objects begin and end (i.e., stairs), clutter should be minimized, and all necessary objects should be visible and always in the same place (Forse, 1994).

PSYCHOSOCIAL IMPLICATIONS

The viability of a program to implement home modifications depends on the receptivity of the client (Rossi & Freeman, 1989). Barriers to the implementation of home modifications persist even when there are no constraints due to lack of information or expense (Glosselin et al., 1993). If this line of reasoning is pursued, it would stand to reason that lack of consumer involvement might lead to dissatisfied customers who do not use devices. Poor aesthetic quality, awkwardness, embarrassment at having to use a device or to make modifications can also negatively effect usage (Gage, Fryday-Field, 1997). The stigma that one may feel due to having a disability could discourage use of devices (Trickey, Maltias, Gosselin, Robitaille, 1993).

Occupational therapists use a client centered approach which addresses the whole person. The mind cannot and should not be separated from the body, if interventions are to be truly successful. Krefting and Krefting (1991) agree with current occupational therapy practice models which incorporate the performance context, specifically, those that revolve around cultural concerns with respect to the acceptance and use of equipment by older adults. Using culturally sensitive approaches, the occupational therapist can make the critical difference between whether services are accepted or refused by the client (Barney, 1991).

Satisfaction with the modifications can positively impact a person's ability to cope with the challenges they face (Clemson & Martin, 1996). The literature points to several studies focusing on the use of devices and/or the implementation of modification in the home. Some problems were systems related–revolving around lack of or limited follow up services after discharge, as well as restrictive third party reimbursement policies (Mann, 1997). Other findings indicated that some older adults found modifications too cumbersome, equipment-device failures, cost of incorrect prescription, and/or lack of appropriate instructions, to be problematic (Gitlin, Levine & Geiger, 1993; Gage, Cook & Fryday-Field, 1997). While some elderly indicated that their conditions improved (Parker & Thorslund, 1991), others experienced a deterioration in their physical and/or health conditions. In both cases a cessation in use of specific devices occurred. Clemenson and Martin (1996) found that if older adults believed positive benefits would result from use of a specific device, this perception increased usage. Trickey et al. (1993), looking at home adaptions, speculated that abandonment of home fixtures was due to the fact that permanent fixtures cannot be adapted to ongoing changes associated with aging. They also found that when cost was eliminated, older adults were willing to make use of home modifications. Filion, Wister, and Bobletz (1992) found the elderly over 75 live on a day-to-day basis and give little if any thought to seeking support services and/or making design alterations. These individuals apparently prefer to cope on their own despite difficulties.

CONCLUSION

Once a home safety assessment has been completed and the identified risk factors corrected, sometimes problems are not resolved. Older individuals and their families need to be empowered with the skills to conduct their own periodic reassessments of home safety, to identify emerging needs and use their acquired skills to problem solve solutions (Connell & Wolf, 1997). In the last three decades the body of knowledge on home modifications and adaptions has expanded. With the prediction of a growing elderly population, their desire to "age in place" and maintain independent living, the commitment of many investigators will be needed. Along with this a better understanding of the multiple environmental needs of this population should prompt the creation of reliable and convenient tools to discover acceptable cost effective solutions.

REFERENCES

Aitkens, A., & Finan, W. (1992). *Housing an Aging Population*. Canada: National Advisory Council on Aging.

American Association of Retired Persons. Consumer Affairs/Program Department (1990). *Understanding Senior Housing for the 1990's*. Washington, D.C.

American Phychological Association. (1997). *What practitioners should know about working with older adults*. Washington, DC: American Psychological Association.

Barney, K. F. (1991 July). From Ellis Island to Assitive Living: Meeting the Needs of Older Adults from Diverse Culture. *The American Journal of Occupational Therapy*, 586-592.

Christiansen, C. & Baum, C. (1991). *Occupational Therapy: Overcoming Human Performance Deficits.* New Jersey: Slack.

Christenson, M. & Krantz, G. (1993). EASE Enhancements Adapting Senior Environments. *Technology* (4)5.

Clemson, L., Roland, M., & Cumming, R. (1992). Occupational therapy assessment of potential hazards in the homes of elderly people: An inter-rater reliability study. *Australian Occupational Therapy Journal, 39*(3), 23-26.

Clemson, L., & Martin, R. (1996). Usage and Effectiveness of Rail, Bathing and Toileting Aids. *Occupational Therapy in Health Care*, 41-58.

Clemson, L. (1997). Types of hazards in the home of elderly people. *The Occupational Therapy Journal of Research, 17*, 200-213.

Clemson, L., Roland, M., & Cumming, R. (1992). Occupational Therapy assessment of potential hazards in the homes of elderly people: An inter-rater reliability study. *Australian Occupational Therapy Journal, 39*(3), 23-26.

Connell, B. & Wolf, S. (1997). Environmental and behavioral circumstances associated with falls at home among health elderly individuals. *Archives of Physical Medicine and Rehabilitation, 78*, 179-186.

Cristarella, M. C. (1977). Visual functions of the elderly. *American Journal of Occupational Therapy, 31*, 432-440.

Dahl, R. & Lejnieks, T. (1990). Occupational therapy in environmental planning for the elderly. *Gerontology SISN, 13*, 2-4.

Filion, P., Wister, A., & Coblentz, E. J. (1992, January). Subjective Dimensions of Environmental Adaptation Among the Elderly: A Challenge to Models of Housing Policy. *Journal of Housing for the Elderly, 10*, 3-32.

Forse, D. (1994). Modifying the home environment of the client with senile-dementia of the Alzheimers type. *Home & Community Health SIS 1*(4), 1-4.

Gage, M., Cook, J. V., & Fryday-Field, K. (1997). Understanding the Transition to Community Living After Discharge from an Acute Hospital: An Exploratory Study. *The American Journal of Occupational Therapy, 47*(2), 96-103.

Gitlin, N. L., Levine, R., & Geiger, C. (1993, February). Adaptive Devices Use by Older Adults with Mixed Disabilities. *Archives of Physical Medicine and Rehabilitation*, 149-152.

Golant, S. (1986). Understanding the diverse housing environments of the elderly. *Environments, 18*(3), 35-51.

Gosselin, C., Robitaile, Y., Trickey, F., & Maltias, D. (1992, December). Factors predicting the implementation of home modifications among elderly people with loss of independence. *Physical & Occupational Therapy in Geriatrics, 12*, 15-27.

Hays, C. (1978). General medicine and surgery. In H. L. Hopkins & H. D. Smith (Eds.), *Willlard and Spackman's Occupational (5th edition)*. Philadelphia: J. B. Lippincott Co.

Health and Welfare Canada. (1984). *Help yourself! Hints from the handicapped, minister of supply and services*, Canada.

Hettinger, J. (1995). Falling Down. *O.T. Week*, Sept., 18-19.

Hettinger, J. (1995). A focus on vision. *O.T. Week*, August 10, 20-21.

Hettinger, J. (1996). "Practitioner and architects make a dynamic team that can help older american age in place and even permit some people with disabilities to remain in their own home." *O.T. Week*, July 4.

Kendig, H. (1989). *Directions on ageing in new south wales background*. Sydney: Office on Ageing, NSW Premier's Department.

Krefing, L. H., & Krefting, D. V. (1991). Cultural influences on performance. In C. Christian & C. Baum (Eds.), *Occupational Therapy: Overcoming human performance deficit*. (102-1220). Thorrofare, NJ: Slacks.

LaPlante, M. (1997). The prevalence of need for assistive technology devices and home accessibility features. *Technology Disability, 6*, 17-26.

Lawton, M. P. (1985). The elderly in content: Perspectives from environmental psychology and gerontology. *Environment and Behavior, 17*, 501-519.

Letts, L. (1995). Assessing safe function at home: The SAFER Tool. *Home and Community Health SISN, 2*(1) 1-2.

Letts, L. et al. (1998). The reliability and validity of the safety assessment of function and the environment for rehabilitation (Safer Tool). *British Journal of Occupational Therapy, 61*(3), 127-130.

Levy, L. (1990). Sensory change and compensation. In L. J. Davis & M. Kirkland (Eds.), *Role of Occupational Therapy with the Elderly*. 49-67, Rockville, Maryland: American Occupational Therapy Association.

Levy, S. B., & Gordon, A. R. (1988). Age related vision loss: Functional implications and assistive technologies. *International Journal of Technology and Aging 1*(2), 16-125.

Lindsley O. R. (1964). Geriatric behavioral prosthetics. In R. Kastenbaum (Ed.), *New Thoughts on Old Age*. Springer Publishing Co.

Mann, W. et al. (1994). Environmental problems in home of elders with disabilities. *The Occupational Therapy Journal of Research, 14*(3), 191-211.

Mann, W. (1997 January). Aging and assistive technology use. *Technology and Disability*. 63-75.

Neistadt, M. E. (1990). Critical Analysis of Occupational Therapy approaches for perceptual deficits in adults with brain injury. *American Journal of Occupational Therapy, 44*, 299-304.

Ringwald, E. S. (1988). October on the eve of universal design. *Home, 204*.

Roitman, D. (1993). Age associated percepticol changes and the physical environment: Perspectives on environment adoption. *The Israel Journal of Occupational Therapy 2*, E14-E27.

Seelman, K. D. (1990). Communication accessibility: A technology agenda for deaf and hard of hearing people. *International Journal of Technology and Aging, 3*(2) 91-100.

Shamberg, S. & Shamberg A. (1996). Blueprints for independence. *O.T. Practice*, June, 22-29.

Smith D. B. D. (1990). Human factors and aging: An overview of research needs and application opportunities. *Human Factors, 32*, 509-526.

Smolarkiewicz, J. (1998). Smoothing the way in and out. *O.T. Week On Line Feature,* May 14.

Speechley, M., & Tinetti, M. (1991). Falls and injuries in frail and vigorous community elderly persons. *Journal of American Geriatric Society, 39,* 46-52.

Stuen, C. & Offner, R. (1999). A Key to Aging in Place: Vision Rehabilitation for Older Adults. *Physical & Occupational Therapy in Geriatrics, 16*(3/4), 59-77.

Tinetti, M. E., Baker D. I., Garrett, P. A., Gottschak, M., Koch, M. L., Horwitz, R. I., & Yale. (1993). First Trial: Risk factor abatement strategy for fall prevention. *Journal of American Geriatric Society, 4,* 315-20.

Tideiksar, R. (1986). Preventing falls: Home hazard checklist to help older patients protect themselves. *Geriatrics, 41,* 26-28.

Trickey, F., Maltias, D., Gosselin, C., & Robitaille, Y. (1993). Adapting Older Person's Homes to Promote Independence. *Physical & Occupational Therapy in Geriatrics. 12*(1), 1-14.

Trombly, C.A. (1983). Environmental evaluation and community reintegration. In C. A. Trombly (Ed.), *Occupational Therapy for Physical Dysfunction* (2nd edition). Baltimore: Williams and Wilkins.

Walker, J. E., & Howland, J. (1991). Falls and fear of failing among elderly persons living in the community: Occupational therapy intervention. *American Journal of Occupational Therapy, 45,* 119-122.

Wright, S. (1997). The quick fix: Temporary Home Modifications for Persons with Spinal Cord Injury. *Physical Disabilities Special Interest Newsletter, 20*(4), 3.

Zola, I. K. (1993). Aging with a disability. *The Rehab Journal, 9*(2), 3-8.

Index